To Pee or *NOT* To Pee

THE HILARIOUSLY SNARKY **PREGNANCY** ACTIVITY BOOK

PEARL CHANCE TODREEME

ULYSSES PRESS

Published in the U.S. by:
ULYSSES PRESS
P. O. Box 3440
Berkeley, CA 94703
www.ulyssespress.com

ISBN: 978-1-64604-031-5
Library of Congress Control Number: 2020931853

Printed in Canada by Marquis Book Printing
10 9 8 7 6 5 4 3 2 1

Acquisitions editor: Claire Sielaff
Managing editor: Claire Chun
Editor: Renee Rutledge
Cover design: Ashley Prine
Cover art: woman © Elena Pimonova/shutterstock.com; toilet © Pranch/shutterstock.com
Interior design and layout: Jake Flaherty
Interior art: © shutterstock.com

Introduction

How to Use This Book

Well hey there, Preggo! You probably got this book from your baby shower. How was it? Did your mom say something snarky? Did your sister try to steal the spotlight? Was your friend incapable of talking about anything but her recent engagement? I'm sure it was great despite all the little quirks. After all, everyone was there to support you and your baby!

Maybe you've just read that paragraph and are thinking: excuse me, I bought this book for myself TYVM. Well, hey there to you too! It doesn't really matter how or why you've come across this book. What matters is, you're freaking pregnant! Shit! That's big. That's huge. And soon you'll be too.

That's where this book comes in. It will accompany you on your journey through trimesters, as your baby grows from the size of a little tiny seed to a giant fucking watermelon. You'll go through a lot, so it's good that you have this book on hand. It will offer your pregnancy brain (trust us, this is a Thing) a break and entertain you during long Feet-Up Sessions.

You can use this book however you damn well please. After all, it's yours and you're the pregnant one. Most people who get this book in the early stages of their pregnancy start from Trimester 1 and fill it out chronologically. If chronology isn't really your thing, skip around! Do whatever the fuck you want. We support you. There's pretty much no way to go wrong, so adjust your complex and ergonomically designed pillow support structure, tell your partner to get you a freaking pickle sandwich (or whatever your current pregnancy craving is), and get down to entertaining yourself.

And don't forget: you're growing a HUMAN in there. You're the shit!

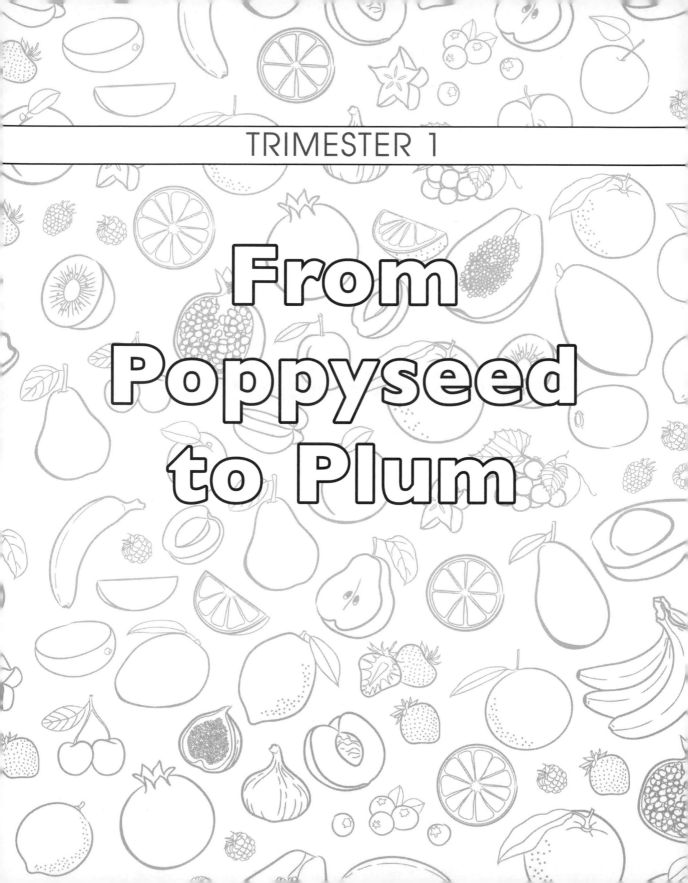

From Poppyseed to Plum

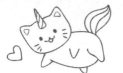

About Me Fill in the Blanks

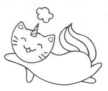

_____. My name is _____.
          (greeting)   (name)

I am _____ years old and pregnant AF. As I fill out this About Me page, I'm feeling
        (number)

_____ , _____ , and
        (emotion)   (emotion)

_____ about being pregnant. It's _____ and
        (emotion)   (adjective)

_____. When I first found out I was pregnant I was in
        (adjective)

_____ and it was _____. At that moment I felt
        (location)   (time of day)

_____, _____, and _____. I told
        (emotion)   (emotion)   (emotion)

_____ about it and they were _____ and said
        (name)   (emotion)

_____! It took us _____ _____ to process, and now
        (exclamation)   (number)   (measurement of time)

we are _____.
              (adjective or emotion)

Some people talk about pregnancy being magical, but I am not a majestic

_____; I am me, and it currently feels like there is a
        (fantastical creature)

_____ in my stomach. I'm dealing with it (circle all that apply):
        (type of food)

A. Pretty well!

B. Okay, but the near-constant war of nerves battling excitement is a bit grating.

C. Badly. Why is there an alien inside me?

D. Fantastically, I actually am a majestic fucking unicorn.

E. There is a monkey banging cymbals together marching around inside my head shouting "you're pregnant" over and over again, so you tell me.

Expectation vs. Reality

Doodle how you envisioned your early-stage pregnant self to look, versus your actual pregnant self:

How I thought I'd look

How I really look

True or False:
The First-Trimester Edition

Let's test your basic knowledge of WTF is up in your first trimester of pregnancy!

1. Your embryo already has teeth. ☐ True ☐ False

2. Your pregnancy was conceived during week one. ☐ True ☐ False

3. Your embryo's heartbeat began before the pregnancy could be detected via ultrasound. ☐ True ☐ False

4. The umbilical cord has one major artery. ☐ True ☐ False

5. Your fetus can "breathe" amniotic fluid. ☐ True ☐ False

6. It's normal to experience a metallic taste in your mouth, almost like sucking on a penny. ☐ True ☐ False

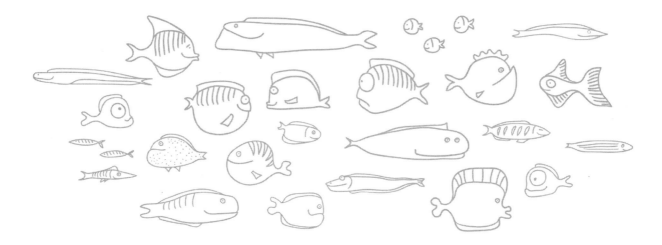

Answers on page 141.

A Valentine for My Valentine

Color in this sweet heart for your sweetheart and tell them, "Thanks for the pregnancy!"

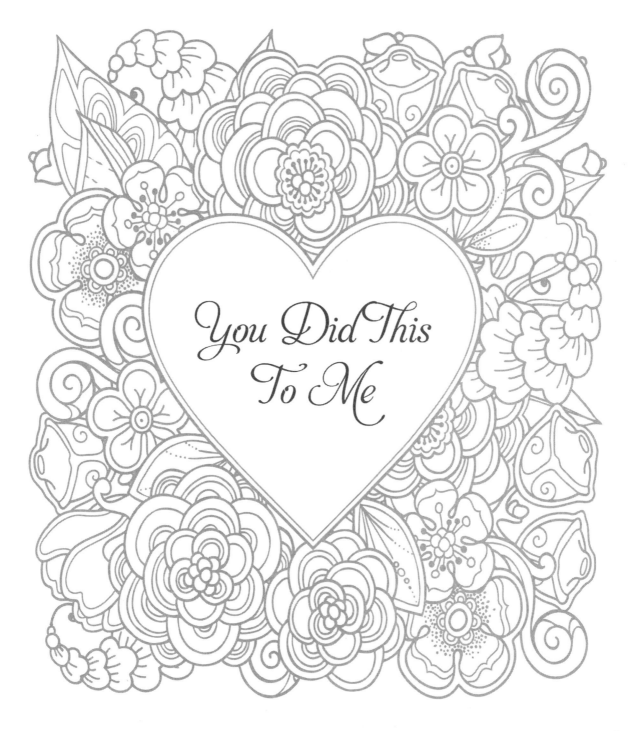

Influencer Life Coloring Page

You could be living in a reconverted panel van road-tripping from coast to coast—but alas—that influencer life is not for you, Preggo. That doesn't mean you can't spend some time coloring in that pipe dream.

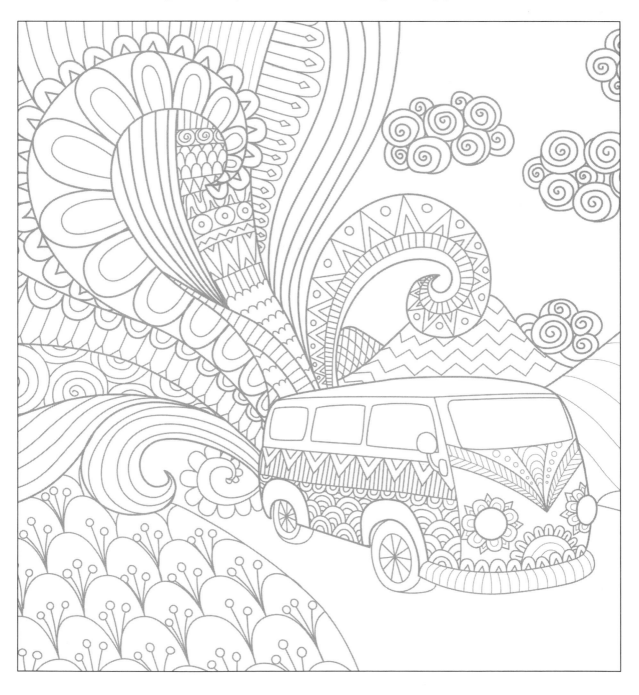

Vision Board for Baby

Pull out all of those random magazines you have in your house, get some scissors, tape, or glue, and get to crafting a vision board for your baby. Do you envision the next Nostradamus popping out of your vag, or perhaps Mother Teresa? Dream big, cut it out, and slap it on this page!

Morning Sickness Word Search

Ahhh, morning sickness. Isn't it fun to suddenly be disgusted by the smells of food you once loved? Isn't it fun to feel nauseous at any and all times of the day—not just mornings? Isn't it fun to be at work and then have to run out of the room with no warning to go yak in the bathroom? Let's explore this joy of pregnancy further with a word search of common triggers.

Broccoli	Onions	Gasoline	Fast food	Red meat
Cauliflower	Fish	Refrigerator	Perfume	French fries
Chicken	Eggs	Deli meat	Toothpaste	Cigarettes
Garlic	Coffee	Bananas	Hand sanitizer	

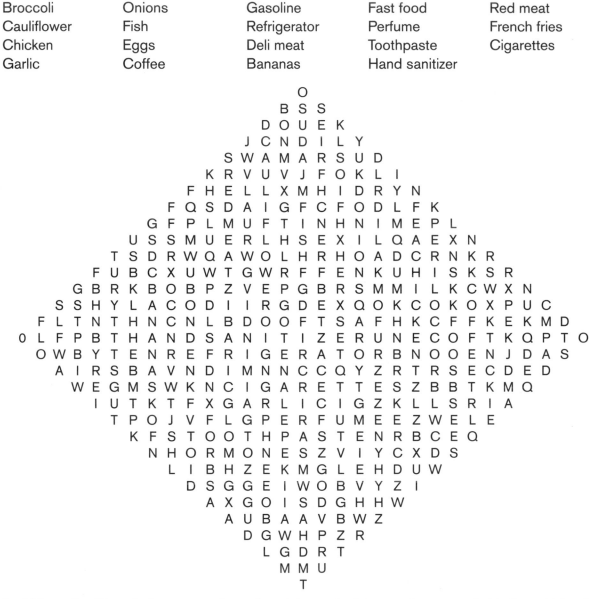

One trivia question: Though the cause of morning sickness isn't known for sure, what is thought to play a role in causing it? Write it here once you've found and circled it: _____

Peeing on a stick and preserving that stick is the start of the many disgusting things you will do as a mother.

Topics to Discuss That Aren't the Fact That You're Pregnant

Waiting until it's okay to tell people about your pregnancy can be the ultimate test of patience. Here are some things to talk about instead of that one thing you really want to be talking about.

- The weather

- Underrated childhood films

- Whether or not you'd be able to make it in the CIA

- Are hot dogs gross or delicious...or both?

- Are Pop-Tarts lasagna?

- Is cereal soup?

- Favorite conspiracy theories

- Favorite random facts

- Should people be allowed to put pineapple on pizza?

- What secret society would you be president of?

- Magical creatures

- The most recent rainbow you've seen

- A product you saw at the grocery store that made you go, "huh."

- What was the first person who ate a lobster thinking?

- The celebrity you'd definitely be BFFs with

- Knowledge gaps

- Doppelgangers

- Memes

- What the youths are up to these days

- Travel

- Family tall tales that definitely aren't true

- Serial killers and/or cults

- The best flowers and the worst flowers

- "What about you, what have you been doing?!"

- Underrated songs

- Your thoughts on the keto diet

- Things your mom told you during your most recent phone call

- The fact that you're freaking PREGNANT—oh wait...not that one!

I'm Fine with Water Crossword

Use the recipes as clues to fill out the crossword puzzle, which is themed around all of the delicious alcoholic beverages you are no longer allowed to drink. Feel free to tear out this page and bring it with you to happy hour, a birthday party, New Year's Eve, or any other occasion where you'll definitely be the only sober person in attendance. While everyone around you gets steadily more and more shitfaced, you can have just as much fun with this crossword puzzle. You're welcome!

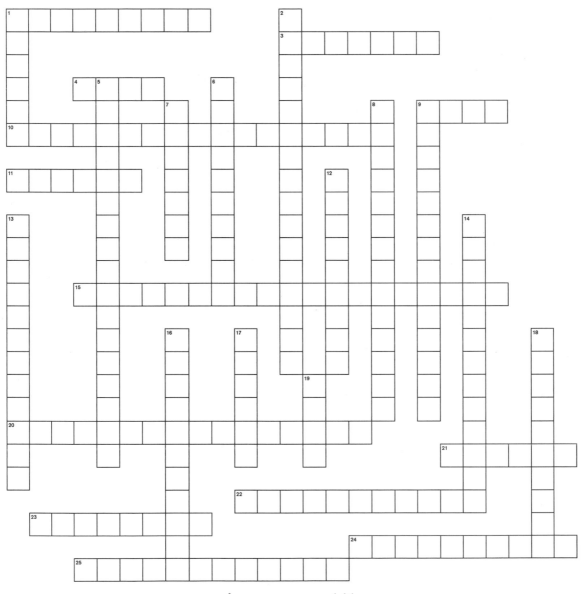

Answer on page 141.

Across

1. Historically made from corn mash

3. A digestif, of life

4. Traditionally sipped from a sakazuki

9. Clear, colorless beverage made from rice, wheat, or barley

10. A one-way ticket to blackout city

11. Amaretto, Kahlúa, Baileys

15. Hemingway's concoction of absinthe and champagne

20. A drink associated with both WWII and tiki bars

21. The world's best-selling spirit

22. Jägermeister, Schnapps, Crown Royal, cranberry vodka

23. A trio cocktail made from whiskey, coffee liqueur, and Baileys Irish cream

24. Vodka and tomato juice, among other ingredients

25. Bright Eyes, turned 21

Down

1. Coming from the heart of the agave plant

2. White rum, cognac, triple sec, and lemon juice

5. Vodka, rum, gin, tequila, sweet and sour, lemon lime soda, and blue curaçao

6. Vodka and cherry liqueur, on ice

7. Italian liqueur made from the seeds of an evergreen tree

8. Gin, sweet vermouth, orange juice, and triple sec

9. A layered shooter with sambuca and Baileys Irish Cream

12. A layered shooter of coffee liqueur, Midori, and Baileys Irish Cream

14. Vodka, peach schnapps, orange juice, and cranberry juice

13. Cherry water, in German

16. Ginger beer, bitters, and dark rum

17. The first Chinese liquor to be produced in large-scale production

18. Rum, pineapple juice, cream of coconut, and orange juice

19. Aka honey wine

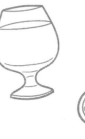
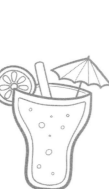
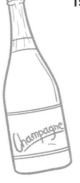

You're WHAT?!

Hold in your mind the visage of the first person you told about your pregnancy. Perhaps it was your mom, perhaps your partner. Maybe it was the harassed mail carrier who just wanted to continue on their route, thank you very much. Maybe it was your Starbucks barista whom you suspect of spelling your name wrong on purpose just for the laughs. Whomever it was, picture their reaction in your head and attempt to draw it below.

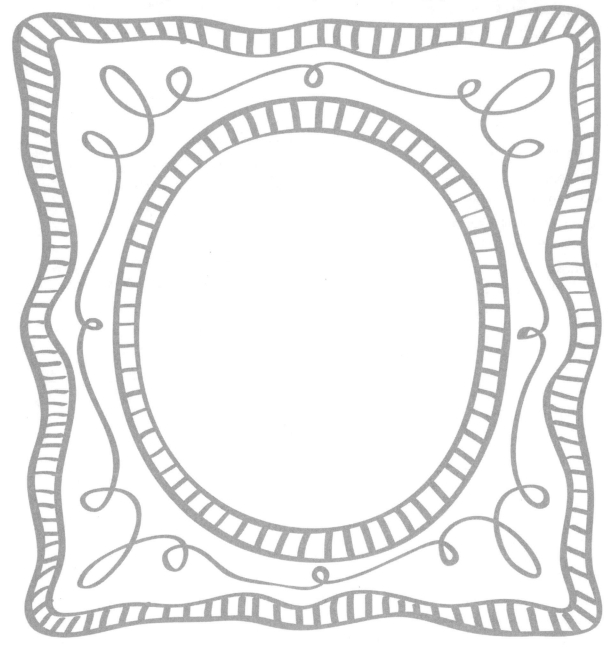

Dream Baby Shower Guest List

Compile the guest list for the ultimate baby shower, including anyone with whom you would absolutely love to celebrate the fact that you got knocked up. It doesn't matter if they're dead or alive—from Jane Austen to Randy from SYTTD, *invite whomever you'd like. It's your party!*

Sudoku Boredom Buster

	7			2		9		
	4		8		6			
	1	2				3		
						8	7	
	6		9	7	2		5	
	2	5						
		1				2	9	
			5		4		3	
		7		6			1	

Answers on page 141.

Would You Rather: Baby Girl Names Edition

Are you the type of person who's had their firstborn's name picked out since kindergarten? Are you completely the opposite of that type of person? Regardless of which type you are, you've probably been asked the dreaded Naming Question many, many times. You've probably gotten some unsolicited (and possibly shitty) advice. You've probably been reminded by Grandma that Great Aunt Prune Mildred Millicent was truly a lovely person and would be a great namesake for your unborn child. Well, if you're going to have to deal with ugly names, why not have some fun with it?

Begin this Would You Rather game by circling your first pick. Then, as you move down the list, fill in the blanks with your top choice from above until the very end. (If your name or the name you've chosen for your child is on this list, sorry not sorry. Just remember: beauty is in the eye of the beholder...or whatever.)

Bertha or Ermegarde

_____ or Abstinence

_____ or Sue

_____ or Baby Yoda

_____ or Amalaberga

_____ or Gertrude

_____ or Banshee

_____ or Drusilla

_____ or Katniss

_____ or Oaklynn

_____ or Bebe

_____ or Cinderella

_____ or Fannie

_____ or Sunilda

_____ or Candy

_____ or Gladys

_____ or Morticia

_____ or Barbie

_____ or Paiyslee

_____ or Kynlee

_____ or Delta

_____ or Renesmee

_____ or Tinsel

_____ or Lakynn

_____ or Bellini

_____ or Dory

_____ or Electra

_____ or Jezebel

_____ or Gazelle

_____ or Mystery

Congrats! The name you've circled at the very end is the name of your brand-spankin'-new baby girl! Let's fill out that birth certificate!

Would You Rather: Baby Boy Names Edition

See directions on page 23 if you're confused.

Hannibal or Fang

_____ or Nym	_____ or Egeus
_____ or Peeta	_____ or Cliff
_____ or Aidoingus	_____ or Algernon
_____ or Betelgeuse	_____ or Farnobius
_____ or Rasputin	_____ or Cymbeline
_____ or Brutus	_____ or Gollum
_____ or Turbo	_____ or Ichabod
_____ or Gunner	_____ or Barnaby
_____ or Puglsey	_____ or Valkamir
_____ or Rutherford	_____ or Ender
_____ or Elmo	_____ or Santa
_____ or Bilbo	_____ or Dracula
_____ or Kace	_____ or Jaeger
_____ or Jax	_____ or Pertruchio
_____ or Lefou	_____ or Bill Nye
	_____ or Peeves

Congrats! The name you've circled at the very end is the name of your brand-spankin'-new baby boy! Let's fill out that birth certificate!

Pregnancy Playlist

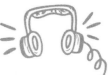

Being pregnant is stressful AF. Sometimes you just gotta say goodbye to your eardrums and blast some music to take your mind off things. Write down your current favorite bops and bangers below.

Try Not to Barf

Hey! You! Barfy McGee! Isn't it funny how they call it "morning sickness" when it's really an all-day-long sort of thing? (Though more accurate, "I have sickness" sounds a bit more ominous than "I have morning sickness.") Wouldn't it be nice if you could just disappear your upset stomach like it's a spy in a hostile war zone? Well, you can't. Instead, try the options we've compiled for you below. May the force to resist your gag reflex be with you.

❑ **Toast**—It's the feast of queasy queens everywhere for a reason. Make sure it's dry or has only a bit of butter on it. Now is not the time to get creative!

❑ **Crackers**—The perfect bland snack to keep your blood sugar interested without releasing the Kraken (aka your gag reflex).

❑ **Preggo pops**—It's not proven that these work every time, but what have you got to lose (besides your last meal)?

❑ **Ginger**—Ale, tea, candies, etc. Keep ginger things in your car, your purse, your desk, and your house. Become the granny you were destined to be.

❑ **Water**—Drinking water is always important. But for morning sickness, try drinking some super-cold water and even chewing on some ice.

❑ **Eat like a little bird**—Make this your new mantra: ommmmm, smallllllll, freeeeeequent meeeeeeals.

❑ **Eat before getting out of bed**—In the morning, try to have some crackers or a granola bar before even getting up. Pretend like it's breakfast in bed, lol!

❑ **Eat before going to bed**—At night, try having a protein bar right before going to sleep.

❑ **Cold food**—Try eating cold foods, like applesauce and fruit, that don't have triggering smells.

❑ **Dress yourself in a sack**—Some women experience less nausea when they're wearing loose-fitting clothing. Might as well embrace the maternity tent early on.

❑ **Night glow**—Computer monitors flicker at a rate that could trigger nausea. Try keeping the warmer, darker glow of night mode on all day, and try taking screen breaks if you start feeling sick. And if you get weird looks, just say, "Sorry boss! Don't want me yakking at my desk, do ya?"

Record what scents trigger your nausea, and avoid them like the plague.

What Can You Smell?

That pregnancy nose really hits differently. Are you feeling like you could join the canine bomb squad and sniff out illegal substances at the airport? List the top five things you can smell with your newfound first-trimester nose that you never could have detected before you were pregnant.

1. _____

2. _____

3. _____

4. _____

5. _____

Cool Off!

Hello, you are a walking furnace. First trimester often comes with feeling like you're Mister Heat Miser in the flesh. Here are some tips for cooling off when the option to simply take off all of your fucking clothes and breathe fire is not possible.

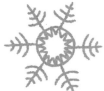

- **Cold washcloths**—Keep a stack of damp washcloths in the fridge (in Tupperware) and use them on the back of your neck. Or, make a new one every time. Just make sure to wring out the cloth thoroughly so it isn't dripping everywhere.

- **Swim**—If your gym has a pool, try swimming as your workout instead of your usual go-to.

- **Breathable fabrics**—No polyester for you, sweaty! Try linen, cotton, and other fabrics that will let your skin breathe.

- **Layers**—If the weather is cool, layer up. That way you can strip as you need to, without the rude awakening that you actually don't have a shirt on underneath your sweater when you go to take it off.

- **Become a vampire**—In other words, avoid being outdoors when the sun is at its highest point.

- **Lie down**—If possible, use the break room or common areas for a quick lie-down, and put your feet up to avoid swollen legs while you're at it.

Forbidden Coloring Page

You can't drink it, so why not color it in? It's almost as good, right? RIGHT?!

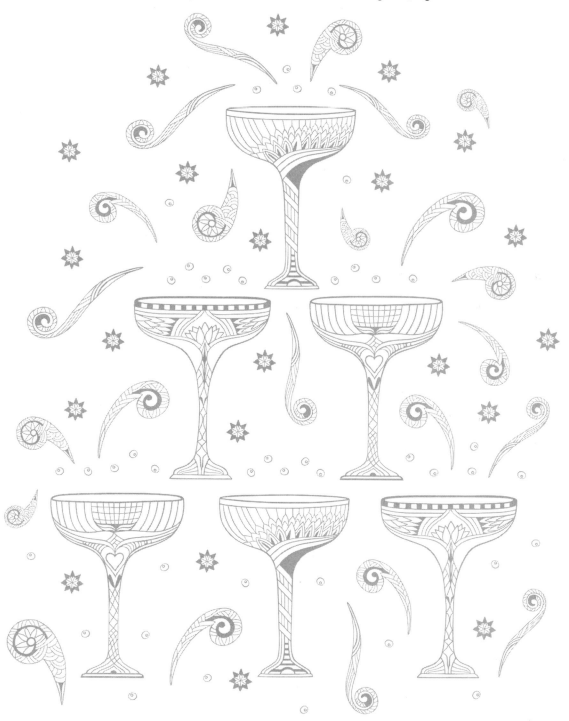

Pregnancy Symptoms Word Search

Find the pregnancy symptoms listed below in the word search, and circle them when you find them. Whew. If you can handle all this shit, you are the definition of a badass!

```
H  U  X  G  Y  G  P  Y  D  B  S  F  E  F  D  G  D  A  V  K
I  B  Q  C  Y  N  F  E  Z  O  Z  E  O  U  N  F  X  V  U  S
G  Y  W  M  T  I  N  B  E  Y  I  O  H  I  I  A  M  D  C  A
H  Y  B  A  I  T  Q  C  M  I  D  R  T  C  H  N  I  L  U  L
E  U  G  Z  L  T  C  A  W  A  N  I  E  F  A  Z  K  K  F  I
R  F  T  T  I  O  K  D  V  X  M  G  R  P  Z  K  P  X  M  V
T  P  F  F  B  P  T  E  Q  O  U  P  A  I  D  S  C  H  E  A
E  Y  B  M  A  S  R  D  V  U  Q  L  N  L  E  E  D  A  E  T
M  M  G  G  T  S  B  O  O  B  N  E  L  L  O  W  S  V  B  I
P  W  C  C  I  Q  Y  X  F  G  S  V  P  W  Z  T  Q  S  V  O
E  I  F  O  R  X  H  A  Z  S  A  P  B  J  L  K  S  F  I  N
R  N  N  P  R  A  T  E  X  E  I  X  Q  N  W  I  G  Q  F  M
A  S  P  S  I  I  V  S  R  N  S  E  H  C  A  D  A  E  H  G
T  O  Z  I  G  W  E  I  K  M  O  O  D  C  H  A  N  G  E  S
U  M  A  U  X  F  R  N  B  L  O  A  T  I  N  G  X  O  U
R  N  E  Z  J  H  A  K  X  G  A  E  S  U  A  N  M  F  V  D
E  I  Q  P  M  D  E  S  C  F  S  I  L  R  K  G  I  G  H  D
K  A  Z  L  S  X  O  O  V  Q  X  Y  Q  O  N  F  S  W  K  S
E  Z  R  I  F  A  F  Z  J  E  L  J  G  U  D  Z  S  X  P  K
E  G  M  F  M  L  G  R  L  R  M  C  T  D  D  E  N  C  Y  G
```

Spotting	Dark nipples	Gas	Cravings
Fatigue	Peeing a lot	Dizziness	Missed period
Nausea	Mood changes	Salivation	Irritability
Vomiting	Higher temperature	Headaches	Insomnia
Swollen boobs	Bloating	Backaches	Food aversions

Answers on page 141.

Pregnancy Cravings Word Search

Find these crazy cravings in the word search and circle as many as you can before one of your own cravings takes over and you must make an emergency trip to the grocery store. Who knows...you might even get some delicious inspo.

```
I T E G Q Y N X S P T F B S N W W T A A
C F W N A G K L N U U N M B R R S E N O
E S I I P R I Y A Z N R H I O S Z F C R
C P X B N M D R T W X G Y U C L J S H M
R H F N J K K E D I R T M S D E D C O P
E K X I V R I V T A Y B C Z E Z T Y V S
A Z M P E F Z E V T E C W S N L M M I N
M S D U Z W B Y S K O C J G N O P H E O
T T A H X V O L N W U S U Z A H N A S I
O S I W S N H T K U I E F T C V D K M N
A W Z G F Q K U P V Z T Z W T Z Y B Y O
S Y G R G R Q O B Q Z B H E S E P V X L
T E U N O L E M R E T A W R Y P L V I L
L I C G U O X Z O T C E U T A F O N G T
T M R G O O D B A R S D Q O I N C U G U
K A G W F B E K A H P A O U E P C L Q H
S E L K C I P H L Q P U W X L R E H C O
H X V E K S Y G U X T B H G S S X P A O
I Q C C P P L R D H R G T R X I K D H H
P Q V W Q O M Z J M N Q H K C H N B Y J
```

Gardetto's	Maple syrup	Gravy on fruit	Mr. Goodbars
Ice cream toast	Canned corn	Onions	Anchovies
Watermelon	Slim Jims	Pickles	Lettuce
Eggs	Sauerkraut	Twinkies with ranch	Dirt

Answers on page 142.

I'm growing
a person
inside me.
What are
you doing?

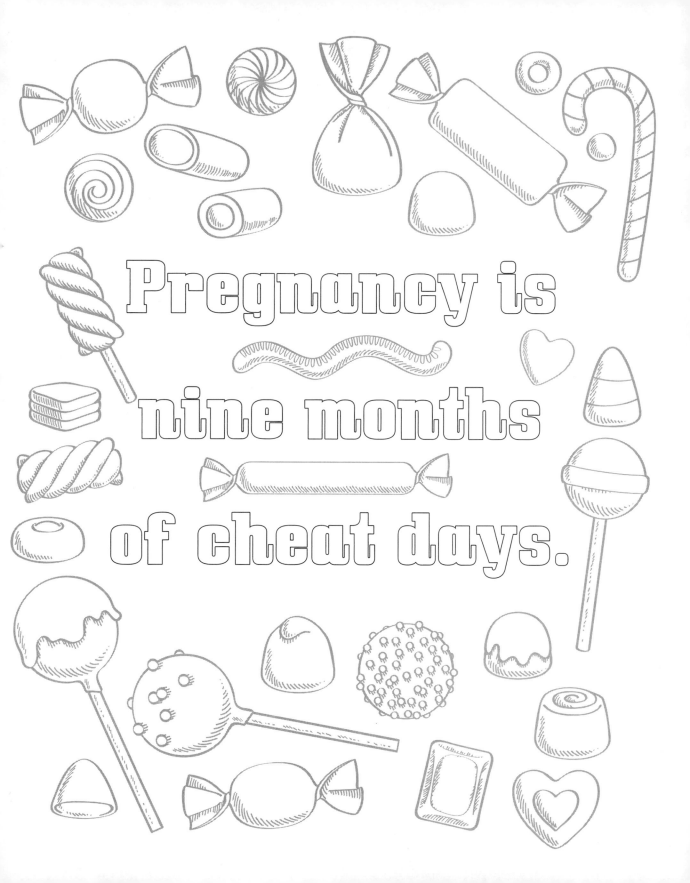

Pregnancy is nine months of cheat days.

Pregnancy:
the time when
you can blame all
of your breakdowns
on hormones.

Journal Time

First-trimester journal time. Write down all of the thoughts going on in that hormone-laden brain of yours. From worries to hopes and dreams to things that are pissing you off, leave nothing out. You'll be happy to have something to look back on once you have that kid!

_____

_____

_____

_____

_____

_____

_____

_____

_____

_____

_____

_____

_____

_____

_____

Baby Store Maze

Get to the checkout with your cartful of excessive purchases for Baby, most of which are completely unnecessary.

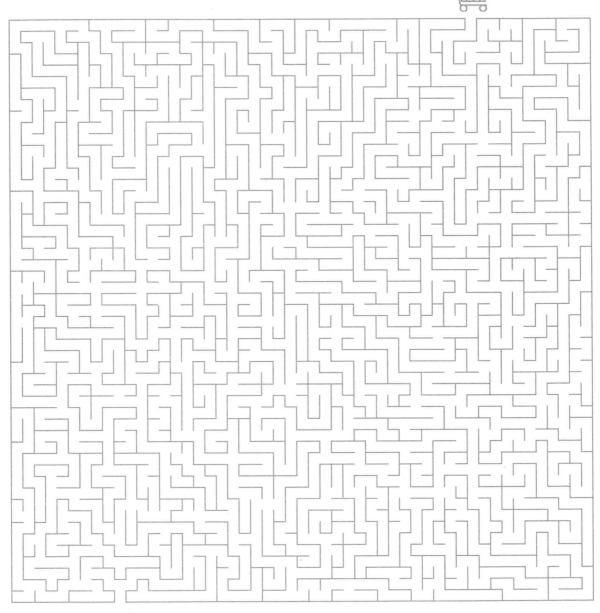

Answer on page 142.

Nursery Rhyme Fill in the Blank

Fill in the missing words from these classic nursery rhymes.

1. Patty cake, patty cake, baker's man. Bake me a cake as _____ as you can.

2. Twinkle, twinkle, little star, how I wonder what you are. Up above the world so high, like a _____ in the sky.

3. Baa, baa black sheep, have you any wool? Yes sir, yes sir, _____ bags full.

4. Hickory dickory dock, the mouse ran up the clock. The clock struck _____, the mouse ran down. Hickory dickory dock.

5. Jack and Jill went up the hill to fetch a _____ of water. Jack fell down and broke his crown and Jill came _____ after.

6. Little Boy Blue, come blow your horn. The _____ in the meadow, the _____ in the corn.

7. Mary, Mary, quite _____, how does your garden grow? With _____ bells, and _____ shells, and pretty maids all in a row.

8. Do you know the Muffin Man, who lives on _____ _____?

9. Ring-a-round the _____, a pocket full of _____. Ashes! Ashes! We all fall down!

10. Three blind mice. Three blind mice. See how they run. See how they run. They all ran after the _____ wife, who cut off their _____ with a _____ knife. Did you ever see such a sight in your life, as three blind mice?

11. Little Miss Muffet sat on her tuffet, eating her _____ and _____. Along came a _____ who sat down beside her, and scared Miss Muffet away.

Answers on page 142.

WTF Are You Thinking about Pie Chart: First Trimester

What is occupying your mind most right now? Fill in this TED talk–worthy pie chart and admire the graphic depiction of the inside of your brain.

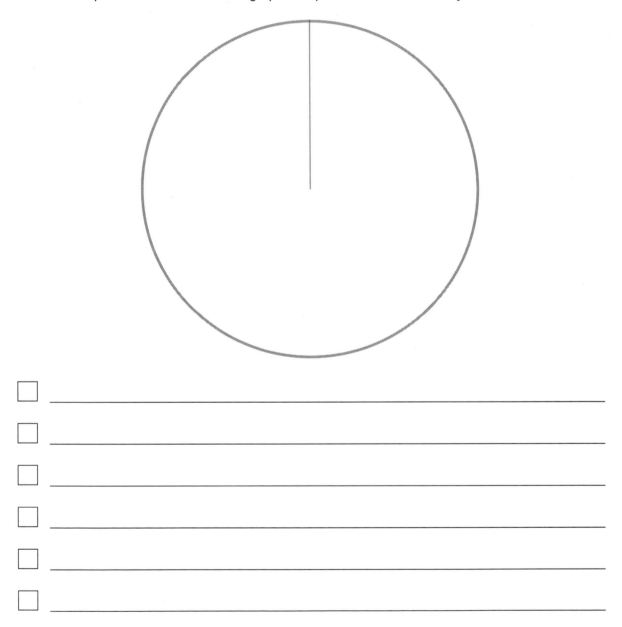

☐ _____

☐ _____

☐ _____

☐ _____

☐ _____

☐ _____

Anxiety-Busting Mandala Coloring Page

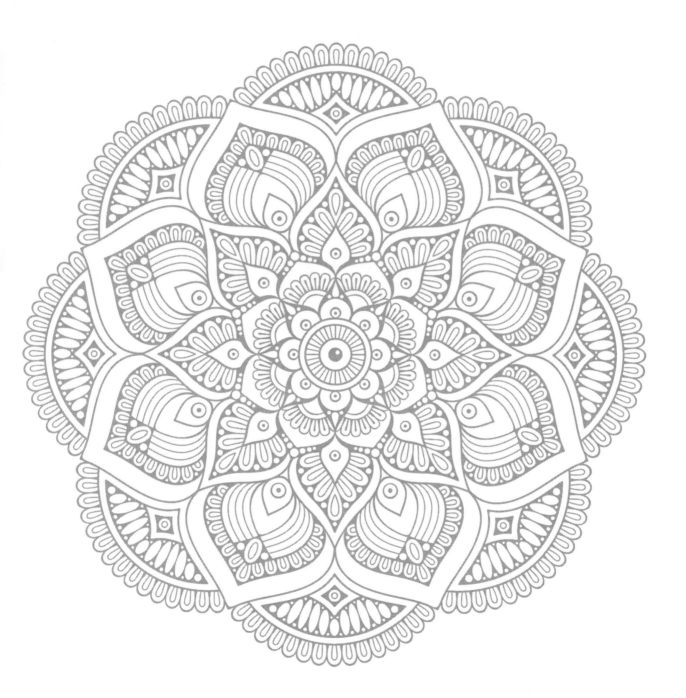

Heartburn Thermometer

Color in these thermometers to represent how much heartburn the corresponding food/drink gives you.

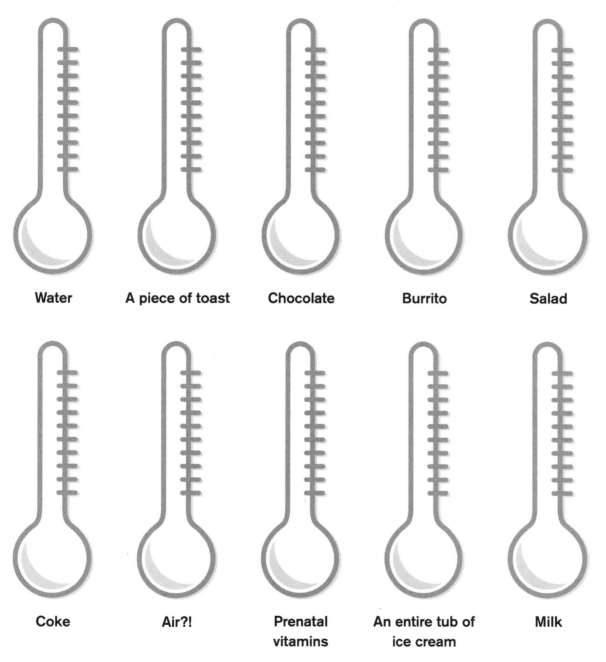

Water

A piece of toast

Chocolate

Burrito

Salad

Coke

Air?!

Prenatal vitamins

An entire tub of ice cream

Milk

Places You've Fallen Asleep

List the top five best places you've caught yourself snoozing, thanks to being bone-fucking-tired every day. After finishing the list, reward yourself with a nice, long nap.

1. _____

2. _____

3. _____

4. _____

5. _____

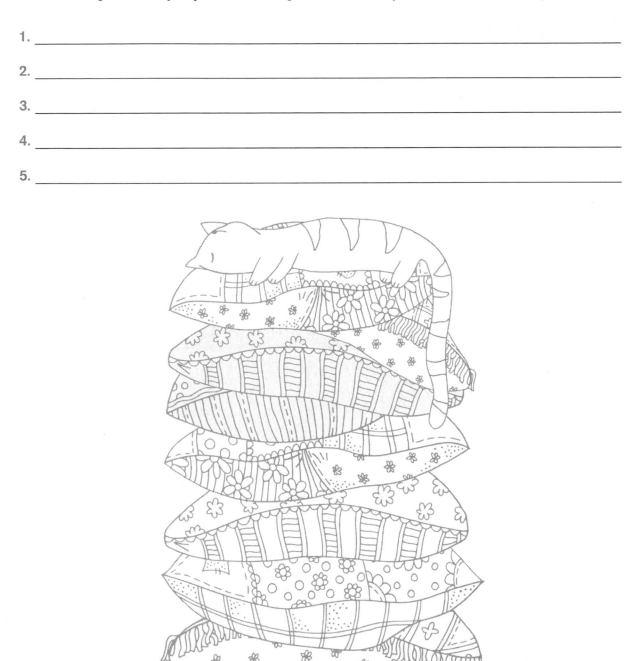

What Should Your Pregnancy Superpower Be?

If you could have a superpower for the nine months you're pregnant, what would it be? The possibilities are endless, but if you need some help getting started, take a look at the suggestions below before writing down your own.

❑ Teleporting to the other side of the room before a stranger can touch your bump

❑ Making morning sickness and nausea disappear

❑ Sleeping through the night

❑ Not having to pee every other minute

❑ _____

_____

❑ _____

_____

❑ _____

_____

❑ _____

_____

❑ _____

_____

❑ _____

_____

❑ _____

_____

From Poppyseed to Plum: First-Trimester Check-In

How are you feeling physically?

_____

_____

How are you feeling emotionally?

_____

_____

What are you thinking about frequently?

_____

_____

What are you excited for?

_____

_____

What are you nervous about?

_____

_____

What was one struggle you've overcome?

_____

_____

What is one of the best memories from this trimester?

_____

_____

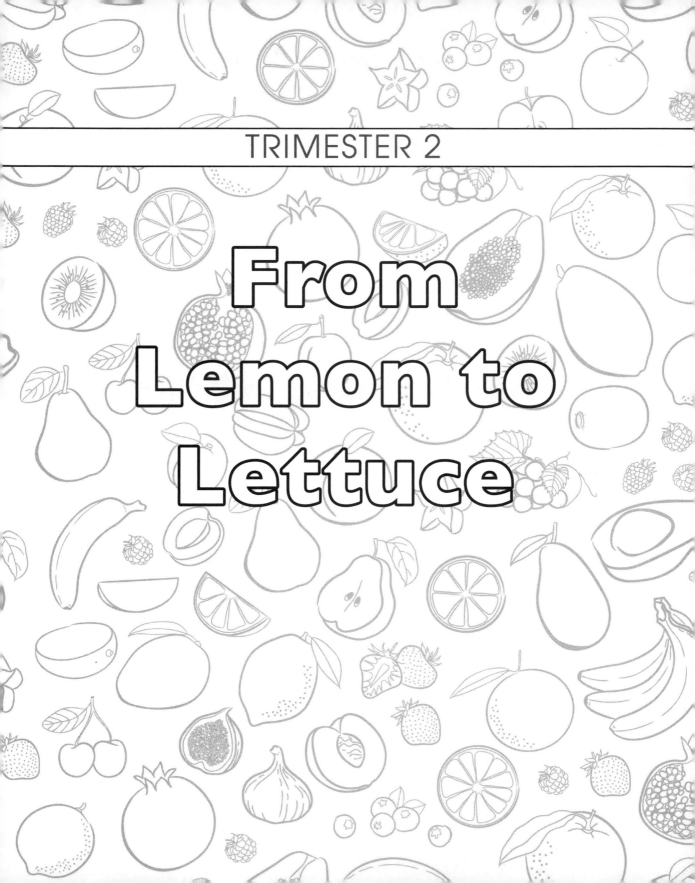

TRIMESTER 2

From Lemon to Lettuce

Expectation vs. Reality

*Doodle how you envisioned your second-trimester pregnant self
to look, versus your actual second-trimester self:*

How I thought I'd look   **How I really look**

True or False:
The Second-Trimester Edition

Let's test your basic knowledge of all the shenanigans currently happening inside your body during your second trimester of pregnancy!

1. The uterus can expand up to 20 times its normal size during the second trimester. ❏ True ❏ False

2. By the end of the second trimester, the fetus measures over a foot in length. ❏ True ❏ False

3. You'll be able to feel the first kicks during the second trimester. ❏ True ❏ False

4. Many women get nosebleeds during the second trimester. ❏ True ❏ False

5. Your boobs have stopped growing by now. ❏ True ❏ False

6. Your baby can start hearing your voice during this time. ❏ True ❏ False

7. You will have sweet, peaceful dreams during this time. ❏ True ❏ False

Answers on page 142.

Nursery Word Search

Find the list of things you'll need for your nursery in the word search and circle them.

```
L  C  X  D  Y  G  O  E  W  T  T  S  D  I  T  Y  O  R  J  O
X  X  H  C  J  M  I  O  F  Z  K  C  N  R  K  E  P  E  Q  L
F  P  T  A  W  C  N  Y  C  E  E  P  A  O  O  T  T  S  L  Z
L  D  L  I  N  Z  X  O  W  B  Z  S  T  G  E  C  N  S  C  K
E  Y  P  W  A  G  X  D  E  N  H  C  W  O  E  E  S  E  C  W
T  E  G  N  P  I  I  E  U  C  B  T  Y  O  T  W  I  R  H  Q
S  J  G  U  O  P  H  N  A  S  T  E  K  N  A  L  B  D  A  Q
R  P  F  H  Q  I  S  N  G  C  L  J  N  E  Y  Y  L  K  I  K
I  N  B  E  A  L  G  Y  Y  T  J  X  Z  A  T  X  S  W  R  Q
M  N  X  B  V  A  K  U  X  B  A  M  S  G  W  P  E  S  C  H
D  U  C  U  J  D  G  S  Y  E  I  B  C  E  S  I  M  E  N  G
I  D  P  Q  B  I  R  C  Q  X  H  N  L  G  I  B  P  V  M  E
M  A  T  T  R  E  S  S  C  O  V  E  R  E  M  H  I  T  V  N
D  V  D  G  P  F  Z  Q  B  B  Y  L  T  Z  A  H  S  B  E  K
P  V  S  A  M  M  M  I  C  Z  G  M  P  F  T  W  B  U  A  O
Z  L  I  R  M  O  Z  H  G  V  Z  S  N  F  T  C  Y  J  L  E
S  D  U  C  M  R  B  N  U  L  D  C  O  S  R  K  Z  S  Z  P
B  U  M  P  E  R  S  I  R  N  A  U  O  Z  E  Q  F  N  P  L
E  X  R  O  W  V  I  U  L  Y  U  E  J  H  S  P  C  M  E  G
Q  X  I  A  B  O  N  B  I  E  X  K  A  T  S  Z  L  B  E  G
```

Crib	Changing table	Bumpers
Mattress	Diapers	Plushies
Mattress cover	Wipes	Mobile
Chair	Trash can	Rug
Dresser	Blankets	Bibs

Answers on page 142.

Do not touch my belly unless you are the one who put the baby in it, or the one who will take the baby out of it.

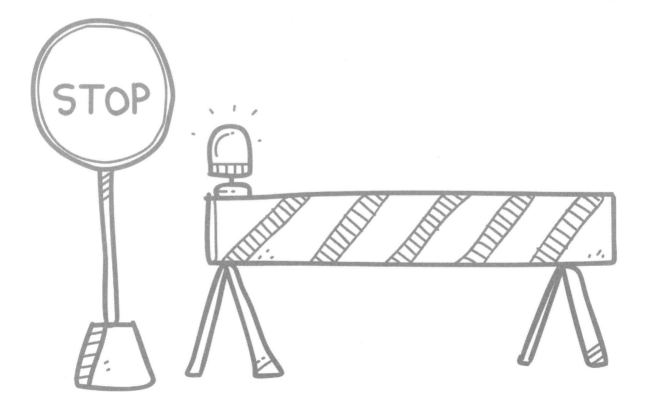

Animal Pregnancy Trivia

Here are some fun trivia tidbits about the animal kingdom that will make you glad (and maybe sad) that you're just a lowly human.

Q: *What mammal is pregnant for the longest?*

A: The elephant. These gentle giants are pregnant for the longest of all mammals. The African elephant is pregnant for a mind-boggling 22 months. Damn.

Q: *What animal (besides humans) spends the most time raising/caring for its young?*

A: The orangutan. These great apes spend almost their entire lives in trees, so it's important for Mom to show Baby the ropes. Mother orangutans spend a whopping six years breastfeeding their babies, and a total of seven years caring for them before they're allowed to go off on their own.

Q: *How do giraffes give birth?*

A: Standing up! Gravity severs the umbilical cord, thanks to an approximate 6-foot drop from vagina to ground. If you're thinking "holy shit, that sounds dangerous," you're right. Sometimes the babies can be fatally injured during this fall, but it's better than the alternative. If a giraffe were to give birth lying down, the baby would most likely be crushed.

Q: *Which animals are able to sperm dump?*

A: Spiders, ducks, and zebra. It sounds gross, but how cool is it that females of these species can say "YOU SHALL NOT PASS" to the sperm deemed inadequate. You go, girls!

Q: *What mammal has the most vaginas?*

A: Marsupials including koalas, wombats, kangaroos, and quokkas. Females of these species have not one, not two, but three vaginas.

Q: *What mammal has the shortest pregnancy cycle?*

A: An opossum's pregnancy lasts for around 12 to 13 days. Must be nice.

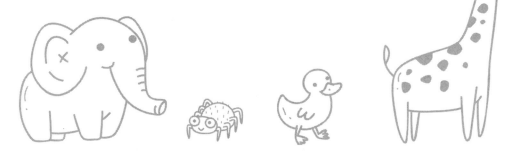

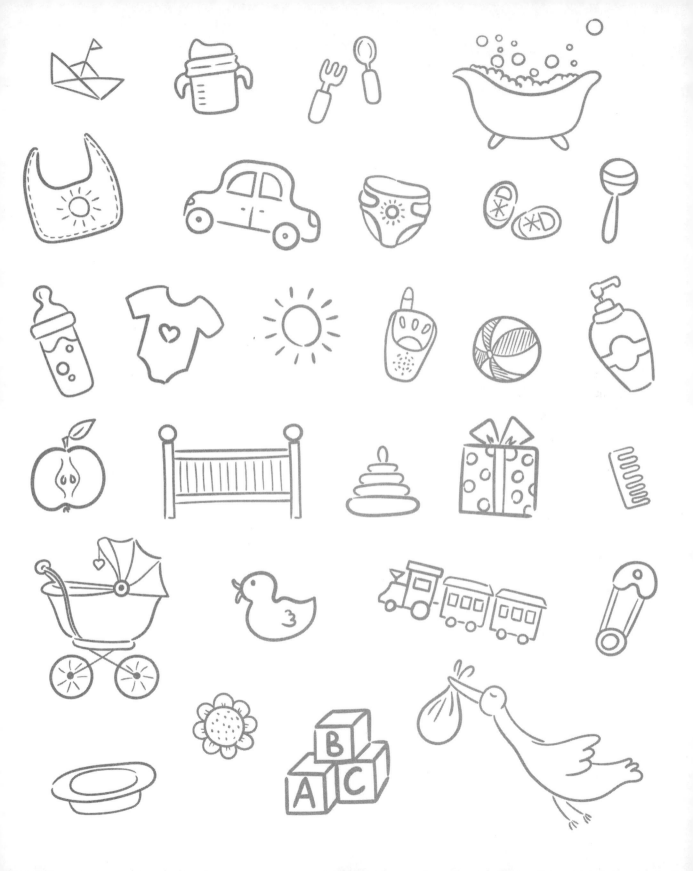

Freaky Things and Fun Places You've Cried

List the top five things you've heard your OB say that were freaky as hell.

1. _____

2. _____

3. _____

4. _____

5. _____

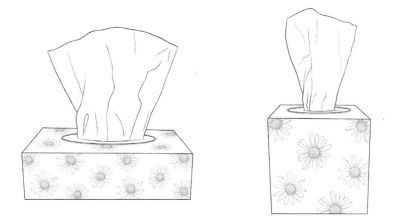

List the top five best and most fun places you've cried, thanks to being pregnant. #Hormones

1. _____

2. _____

3. _____

4. _____

5. _____

True or False: Let's Get Historical

1. In the American colonies, women and midwives both drank beer during childbirth.   ❏ True   ❏ False

2. Painkillers were always available for women during childbirth. For example, during the fifteenth and sixteenth centuries, herbal medicine was used.   ❏ True   ❏ False

3. Doctors and midwives in the 1500s knew what a fetus looked like.   ❏ True   ❏ False

4. Women used to wear corsets through most of their pregnancy.   ❏ True   ❏ False

5. In centuries past, women used to have to share a bed during labor.   ❏ True   ❏ False

6. Taking drugs during pregnancy did not become widely accepted until the 1900s.   ❏ True   ❏ False

7. C-sections (caesarean sections) were named after Julius Caesar.   ❏ True   ❏ False

Answers on page 142.

Congrats on the Boobs

During the second trimester, women usually find that their boobs have—quite frankly—ballooned in size. Celebrate your magical new endowments by writing down every slang term you can come up with for breasts.

_____

_____

_____

_____

_____

_____

_____

_____

_____

_____

_____

_____

_____

_____

Lullaby Fill in the Blank

Fill in the missing words from these classic lullabies.

1. Rock-a-bye baby, on the _____,

When the wind blows, the cradle will _____,

When the _____ breaks, the cradle will fall, And down will come baby,

cradle and all.

2. Hush, little Baby, don't say a word, Mama's gonna buy you a _____.

And if that _____ don't sing, Mama's gonna buy you a

_____.

3. You are my _____, my only _____.

You make me happy when skies are _____.

You'll never know _____, how much I love you.

Please don't take my _____ away.

4. Lavender's blue _____ lavender's green.

When you are king _____ I shall be Queen.

Answers on page 143.

Babymoon Quiz

Take this quiz to find out where you should go on your babymoon.
Then use the key below to figure out your destination.

1. Pick your favorite color:

   A. Blue

   B. Pink

   C. Yellow

   D. Red

2. Pick the thing that would annoy you most:

   A. People who budge in line.

   B. Shouting drunks at a bar.

   C. A child running around a restaurant unsupervised.

   D. Smokers.

3. What stresses you out most about traveling?

   A. The circle of hell that is the TSA security line.

   B. Packing!

   C. Not doing or seeing enough.

   D. Not knowing the language.

4. How would you spend an ideal day on vacation?

   A. Lying. Down.

   B. Seeing the sights and looking cute while doing it.

   C. Doing all the things! Seriously, you have an itemized list.

   D. Taking photos and having fun with your partner.

5. What is the sign of a great vacation?

   A. Coming home tan AF.

   B. Finding the best souvenirs.

   C. Having gotten to know a new culture.

   D. Feeling sad on the day you have to head home.

Mostly A's: Fiji. Say goodbye to whatever college fund you've saved up for Baby, cuz you're gonna blow it all on a beachfront bungalow and it will be #worthit.

Mostly C's: Tokyo. Just think about it. It's the perfect place to visit while childless. From the epically long flight to awesome cultural experiences, you'll be able to enjoy it all without a wailing baby in tow.

Mostly B's: Paris. You'll have a great time taking in the sights, trying to make a beret work for you, and eating as many croissants as humanly possible. Bon voyage!

Mostly D's: Disney World. That's right, it's the most magical place in the world, and great practice for your baby-filled future. You can watch how other parents manage their little ones and take notes on how and when to bribe children with candy and mouse-shaped Rice Krispie Treats.

Would You Rather: Unisex Baby Names Edition

See instructions from page 23 if you're confused.

Christmas or Domino

_____ or Boo

_____ or Moth

_____ or Spike

_____ or Basil

_____ or Abcde

_____ or Jurnee

_____ or Albany

_____ or Beagan

_____ or Happy

_____ or Kindle

_____ or Ever

_____ or Pooky

_____ or Freedom

_____ or Maine

_____ or Ransom

_____ or Calico

_____ or Jazz

_____ or Mercury

_____ or Derby

_____ or Indy

_____ or Hero

_____ or Magic

_____ or Sailor

_____ or Berkeley

_____ or Silver

_____ or Cloud

_____ or Pilot

_____ or Tiger

_____ or Zealand

_____ or Kale

_____ or Fork

Draw! That! Baby!

According to your doctor, or some article you found online, what size is your baby right now? Take a stab at drawing the fruit that is the same size as your baby.

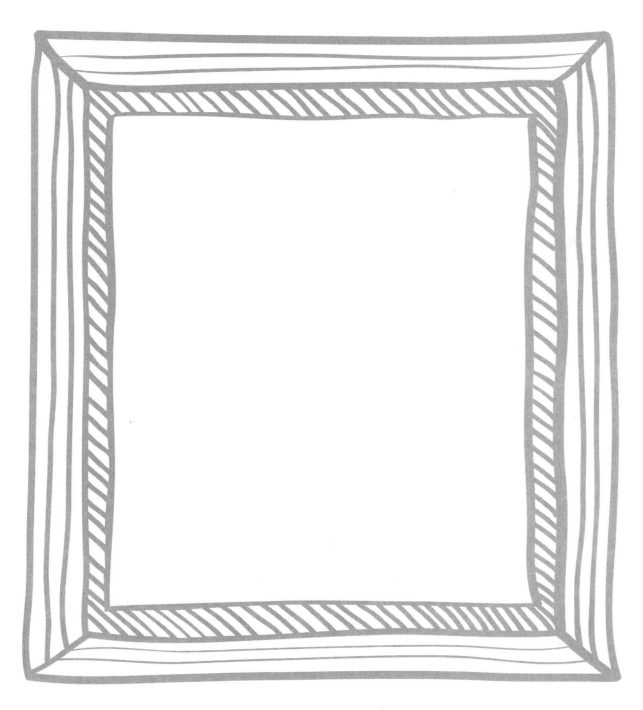

Sudoku Boredom Buster

		3			5			
7					8	1	5	
		1	7	2				8
	1							2
	9						8	
3							4	
8				1	9	2		
	4	2	5					6
			2			7		

Answers on page 143.

Prickly Coloring Pages

Ever wish you could grow some spikes to ward off overly friendly ladies at the grocery store? Here's an appropriately prickly coloring page to entertain you as you indulge in wishful thinking.

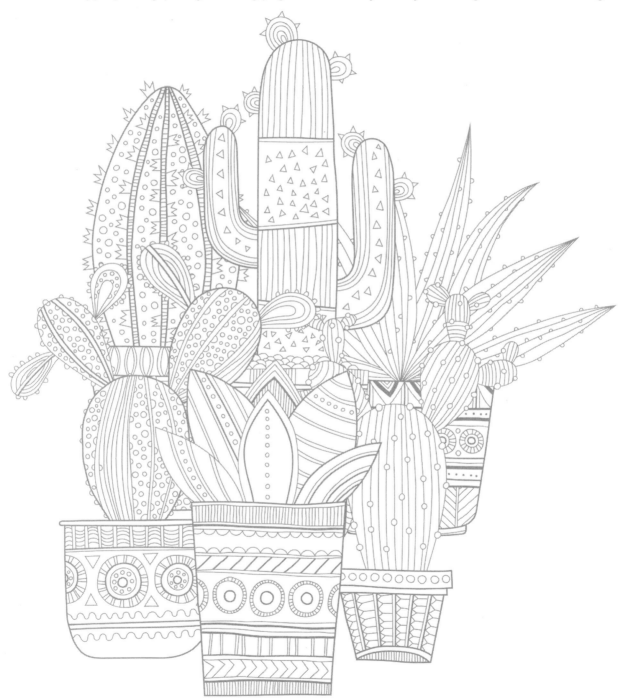

Avoid-the-Unwarranted-Advice Maze

Shit! It was of the utmost importance that you picked up a jar of pickles from the grocery store, but now everyone and their mother are giving you unsolicited advice on how you should give birth to your child. Solve the maze to make it to your car, and try to avoid those know-it-alls!

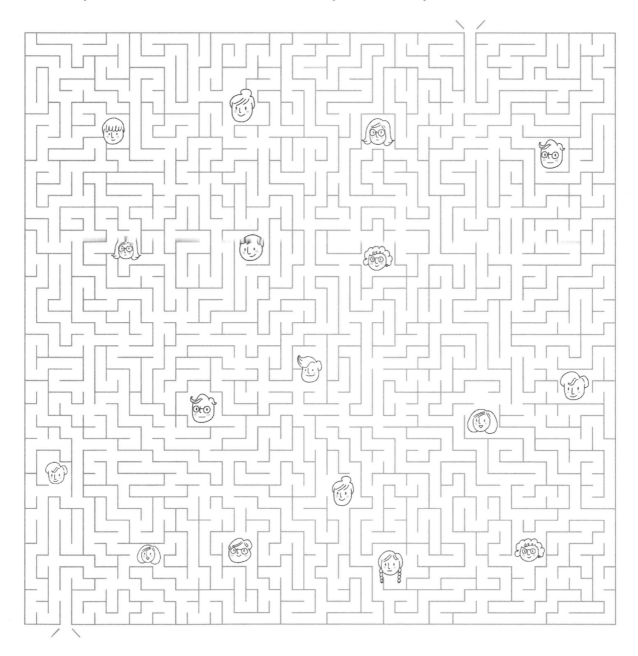

Answer on page 143.

How Many Words Can You Make?

How many words can you make out of the phrase:

Goodbye Morning Sickness?

Write them on the lines below.

_____ _____ _____

_____ _____ _____

_____ _____ _____

_____ _____ _____

_____ _____ _____

_____ _____ _____

_____ _____ _____

_____ _____ _____

_____ _____ _____

_____ _____ _____

_____ _____ _____

_____ _____ _____

_____ _____ _____

_____ _____ _____

_____ _____ _____

Pre-Pregnancy Brain To-Do List

The second trimester is often the time when pregnant women feel the most sane. Let's take advantage of this time of logical thinking and get some shit done. Need to organize the nursery? Put it on the list! Need to create a baby shower registry? Put that on there too!

To do today:

☐ _____

☐ _____

☐ _____

☐ _____

☐ _____

☐ _____

☐ _____

☐ _____

☐ _____

For tomorrow:

☐ _____

☐ _____

☐ _____

☐ _____

☐ _____

☐ _____

☐ _____

☐ _____

☐ _____

Match It Up!

Match up the name to its meaning by drawing a line connecting the two. Stumped?
Flip this page upside down to find the answers.

William	God exists
Benjamin	With gilded helmet
Caleb	Home ruler
Oliver	Son of my right hand
Wyatt	Large, great
Chidi	Whole hearted
Daisuke	Pure, virtuous, divine
Sheng	Brave in war
Apu	Descendant of the ancestor
Enrique	Victory
Nora	Joy of the father
Margot	Hope
Abigail	Light
Lucy	Plum
Penelope	Honor
Kamili	Pearl
Inari	Good feelings
Mei	With a web over her face
Bhavna	Successful one
Esperanza	Perfection

Answers on page 143.

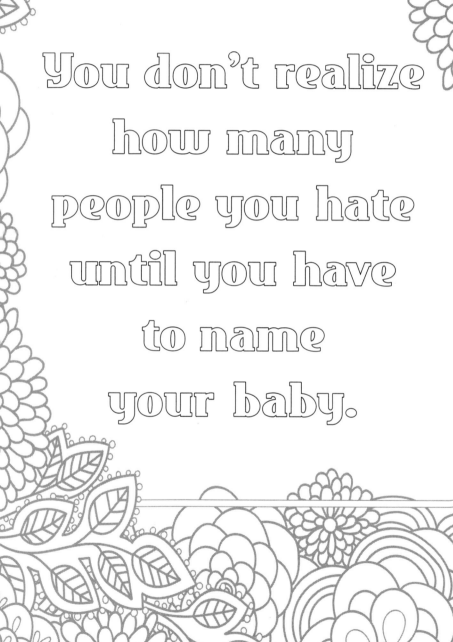

You don't realize how many people you hate until you have to name your baby.

Anxiety-Busting Mandala Coloring Page

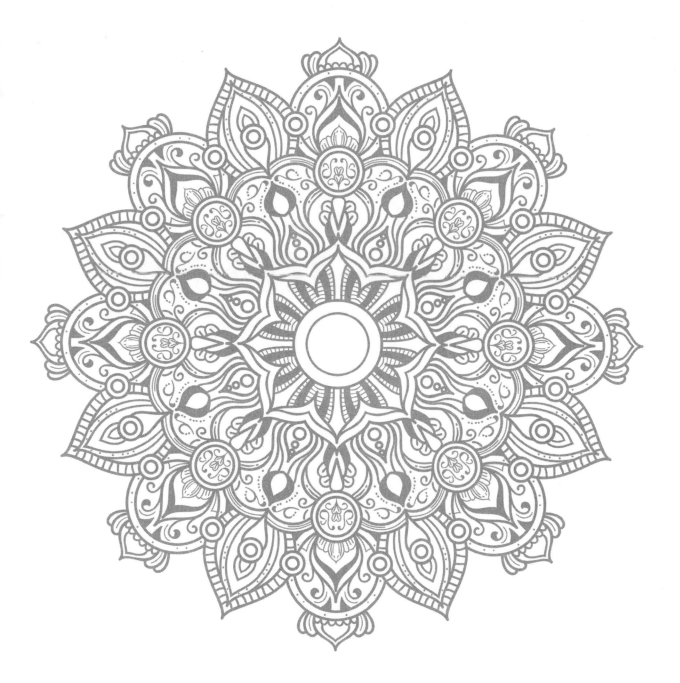

Journal Time

Second-trimester journal time.

_____

_____

_____

_____

_____

_____

_____

_____

_____

_____

_____

_____

_____

_____

_____

_____

_____

Mom Unscrambler

Mom brain: it's that thing when your mom can never remember the names of actors or movies, and you always have to decipher what she means from her descriptions. Well, bad news sister, you're about to have mom brain yourself. Preventative practice below:

1. Mom Name: Lorenzo Dillards   **Actual Name:** _____

Info Mom Knows: "Dates young ladies that are too young for him!"
"Was such a handsome young man."

2. Mom Name: Candy Cumberbatch   **Actual Name:** _____

Info Mom Knows: "Well, she's very famous I suppose."
"I'm not sure about the names of her children, but one is definitely East West."

3. Mom Name: Ice Queens   **Actual Name:** _____

Info Mom Knows: "Those sisters were very sweet."
"The kids love that one song about winter!"

4. Mom Name: Mr. Godfather   **Actual Name:** _____

Info Mom Knows: "Is he in the mafia?"
"Well, he certainly has been in a lot of mobster movies."

5. Mom Name: The Casino Crew   **Actual Name:** _____

Info Mom Knows: "Your father liked this movie."
"There are many famous movie stars in it, probably 13 of them."

6. Mom Name: Elle Worthington Woods **Actual Name:** _____

Info Mom Knows: "She has a whiskey book, an interesting choice in my opinion."
"She really showed her terrible boyfriend who was the better lawyer."

7. Mom Name: Sacramento Sparrow   **Actual Name:** _____

Info Mom Knows: "That young lady from Ireland is in it."
"Also that young man that all the teens follow on Instagram."

8. Mom Name: Dancing Queen   **Actual Name:** _____

Info Mom Knows: "Oh, now this was a wonderful film!"
"If only we could all have Abba as the soundtrack to our lives."

Answers on page 143.

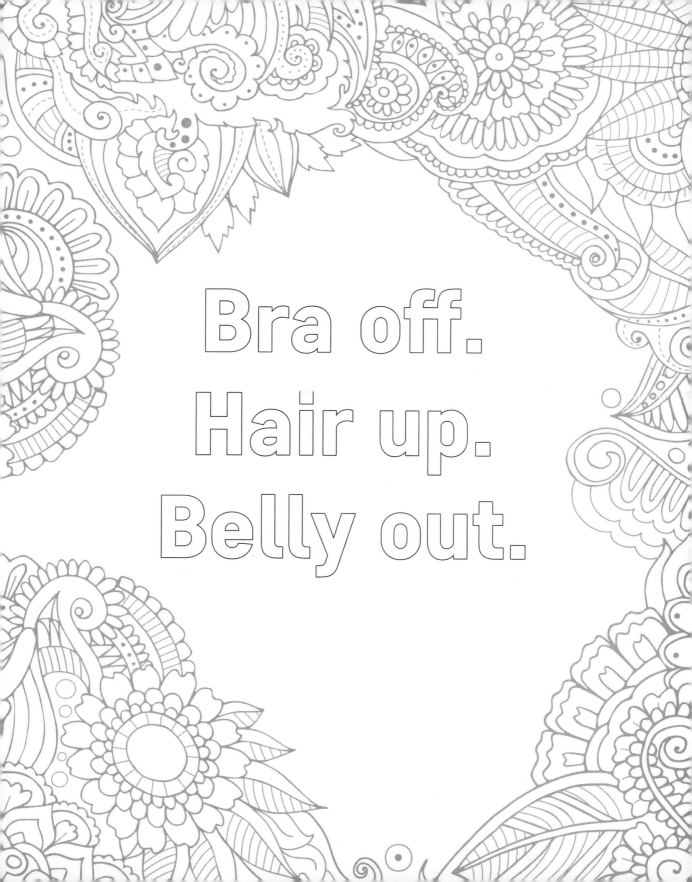

Bra off.
Hair up.
Belly out.

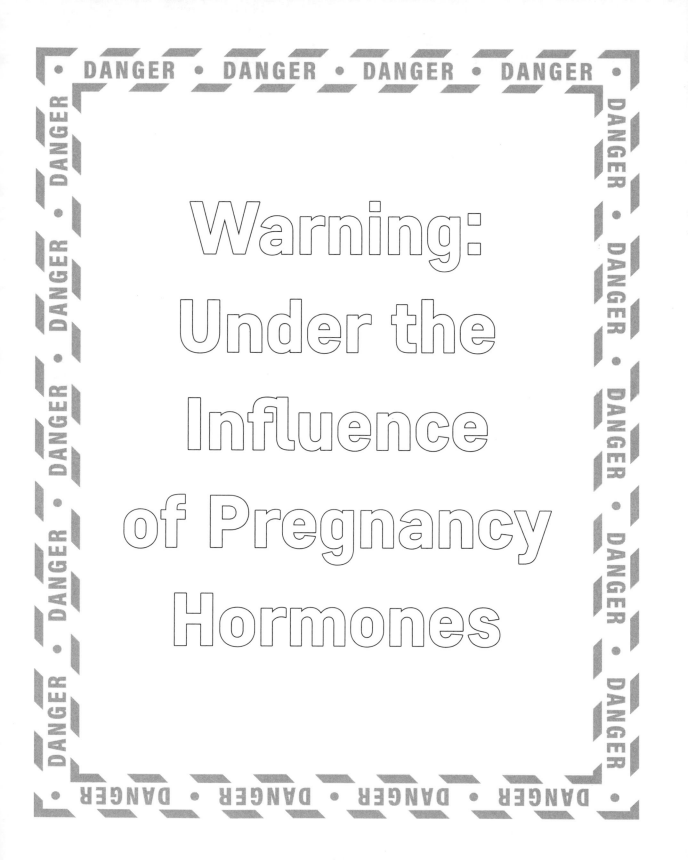

Science Rules! Crossword Puzzle

Let's explore the mysteries of our bodies and the truly insane process of pregnancy and childbirth via a crossword puzzle. Prepare to work those brain muscles (or Google, if you're a cheater!) and have your mind blown by some pretty crazy facts.

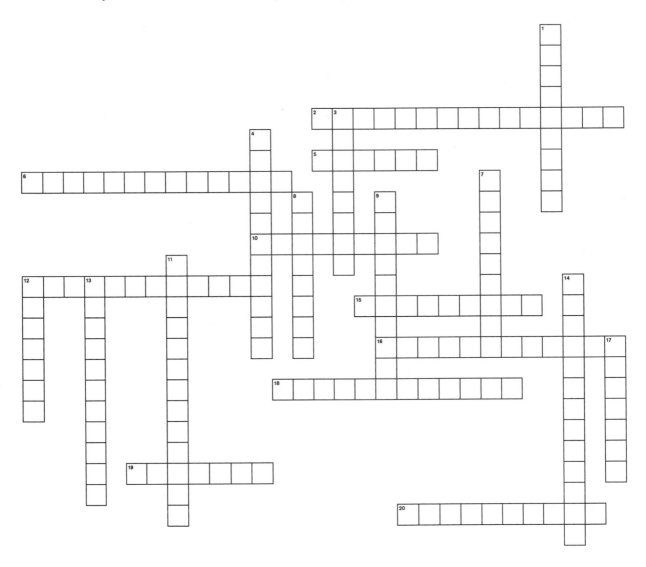

Answers on page 143.

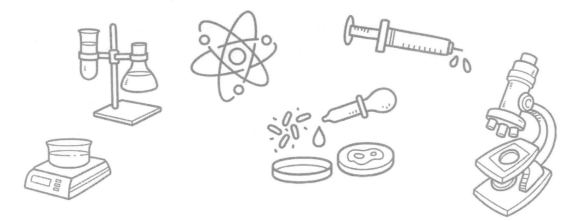

Across

2. One unpleasant, tell-tale sign of pregnancy

5. Another term for a fertilized egg

6. Term for mass of cells during the first 10 weeks

10. The number of times a female has been pregnant

12. A woman in subsequent pregnancies

15. Another word for pregnancy

16. When cells attach to the uterine wall

18. A woman who has never been pregnant

19. The state of an embryo or fetus

20. Pigmentation of the linea alba

Down

1. The period beginning immediately after delivery

3. Hormone released during breastfeeding

4. A woman who is (or has been only) pregnant for the first time

7. A process that stimulates childbirth

8. Provides fetus with nutrients, among other functions

9. Movement in the second trimester

11. Part of a fertilized egg's journey

12. Skin pigment changes

13. A pregnancy is considered term at this many weeks of gestation

14. Connects embryo to placenta

17. This person's rule is a standard way of calculating a due date

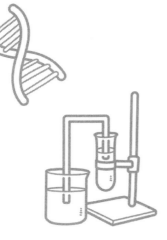

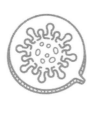

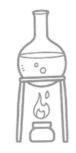

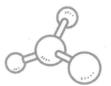

Quiz: Where Should You Have Your Pregnancy Photo Shoot?

1. Where did you spend most of your time before you got pregnant?

    A. At home, lol.

    B. Outside, especially if the weather was nice.

    C. Wherever was cheapest but had food.

    D. At a bar.

2. What is one thing you miss about being not-pregnant?

    A. Not crying at every little thing.

    B. My old body-ody-ody.

    C. Not having smell aversions to very specific foods!

    D. Drinking, duh.

3. What is one thing you can't wait to do with your new baby?

    A. Just having them in my arms! Ahh!

    B. Taking them on vacation!

    C. Seeing their cute reactions to trying solid food for the first time.

    D. Teaching them all of the best bops and bangers.

4. What is one thing you're going to be extra about during this photo shoot?

    A. I just want to be comfortable.

    B. The lighting. I need to be glowing.

    C. Snacks. I do not want to be hangry while modeling my giant stomach.

    D. The glam. My face and my outfits need to be perfect.

5. What is your budget for this photo shoot?

    A. Zero dollars. I'm paying my photographer with homemade baked goods. My photographer is a family member/friend.

    B. Whatever the cost, I'll spend it. I want these photos to look fucking perfect.

    C. It's not big, and half of the budget is dedicated to jalapeno poppers.

    D. I already spent it all on several NECESSARY outfits. Oops!

Mostly A's: Your backyard. You're probably a homebody and you're probably cheap. Nothing wrong with that! Embrace it.

Mostly C's: The buffet. We're just saying, there's nothing wrong with embracing an all-you-can-eat lifestyle while pregnant. Why not show it off during your photo shoot?

Mostly B's: The beach. The wind, the sun, and the sand. Three elements that will make for a bomb pregnancy photo shoot.

Mostly D's: The club. Tell the DJ to put on your favorite song and get some epic mid-motion dance shots. And if someone has a bottle with a sparkler on top, ask to borrow that for a few shots (on the camera, not from the bottle).

Ass-Kicking Activities to Soothe Anxiety

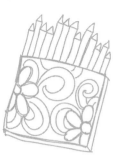

- **Color**

  There are pages in this book for you!

- **Meditate**

  See page 90 for tips.

- **Exercise**

  We don't mean boot camp. Just go for a walk to get your blood flowing again. Moving helps soothe your fight-or-flight response.

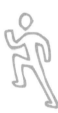

- **Drive**

  If you aren't feeling up for exercise, try taking a drive.

- **Listen to music**

  You have some playlists already written down in this book.

- **Clean**

  Having an organized space can be very soothing to most people

- **Breathe**

  Inhale slowly through your nose, keep your shoulders relaxed. Your abdomen should expand more than your chest. Then, exhale slowly through your mouth by pursing your lips but keeping your jaw relaxed. Repeat.

- **Laugh**

  Watch a show or movie that really cracks you up. Sometimes laughter really can be the best medicine.

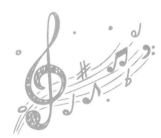

Constipation Station

Color in these constipation cures while waiting for your business to be done.

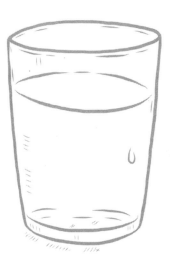

Water

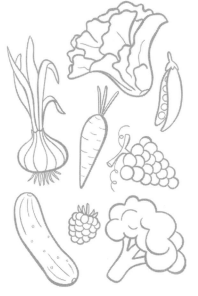

Fresh Produce

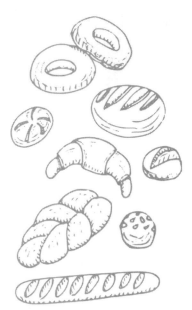

Whole Grains

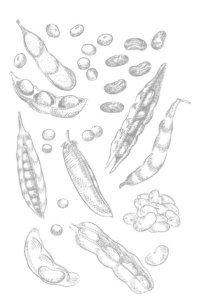

Beans and Legumes

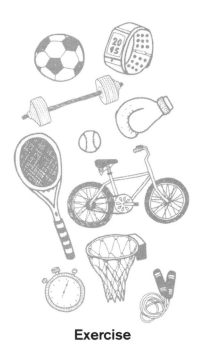

Exercise

Would You Rather?

Choose which scenario you'd rather deal with.

Have swollen sausage legs your entire pregnancy **or**
Have your feet grow an entire shoe size

Have a totally no-nonsense OB **or**
Have an OB who won't stop cracking lame jokes

Be unable to sleep during your entire pregnancy **or**
Be unable to sleep for an entire year after the baby comes

Give up your body pillow during the last few weeks of your third trimester **or**
Have sex during the last few weeks of your third trimester

Be at work and discover your nipples are leaking through your shirt **or**
Be at work and discover there is dried spit up down the back of your shirt

---

Have three strangers come up and caress your stomach **or**
Have three strangers come up and give you unsolicited labor advice

---

Have morning sickness **or**
Sickness coming out the other end

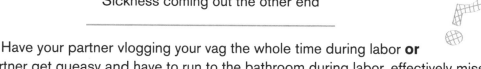

Have your partner vlogging your vag the whole time during labor **or**
Have your partner get queasy and have to run to the bathroom during labor, effectively missing most of it

---

Have post-pregnancy acne **or**
Have post-pregnancy balding

Finish labor and realize you actually had surprise twins **or**
Finish labor and realize your baby is actually the opposite gender of what you'd been told

Dream Journal

Pregnancy can give you the gift of some fucked-up dreams.
Use the space below to write down your top three.

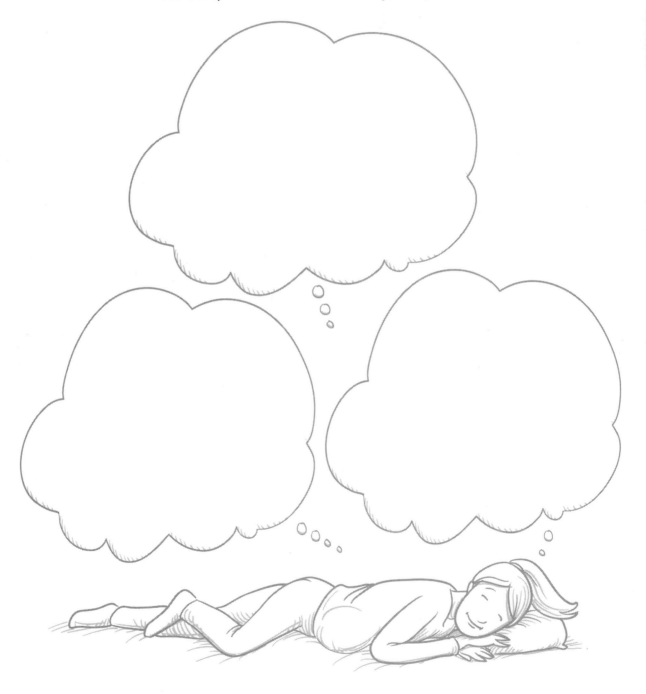

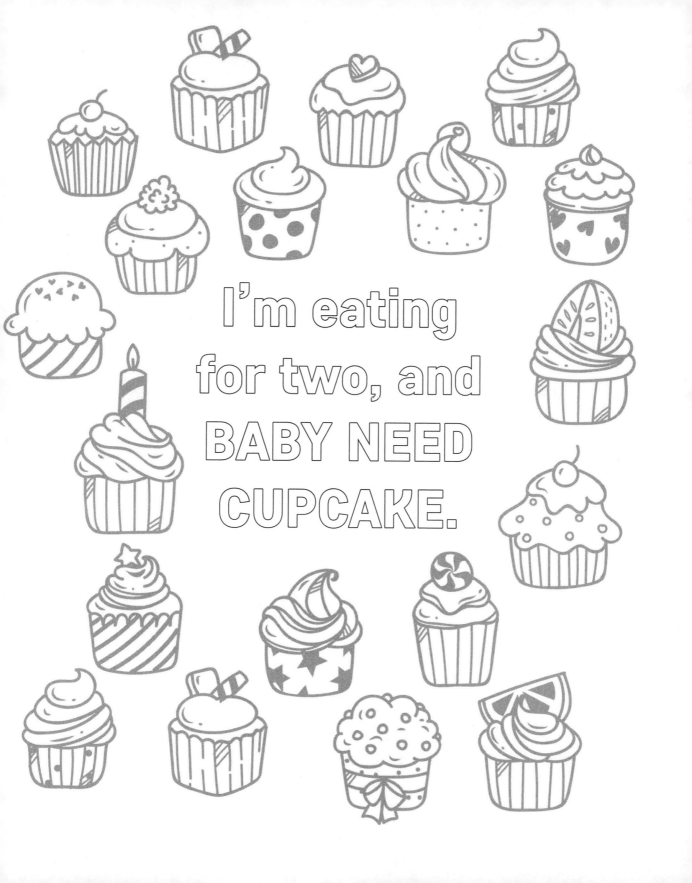

I'm eating for two, and BABY NEED CUPCAKE.

Pin the Dry Skin Patches on the Pregnant Lady

Everyone talks about the pregnancy glow, but no one talks about all those weird patches of dry skin that come out of nowhere. Draw arrows connecting the dry skin patches to the places they've appeared on your body. Just girly things. :)

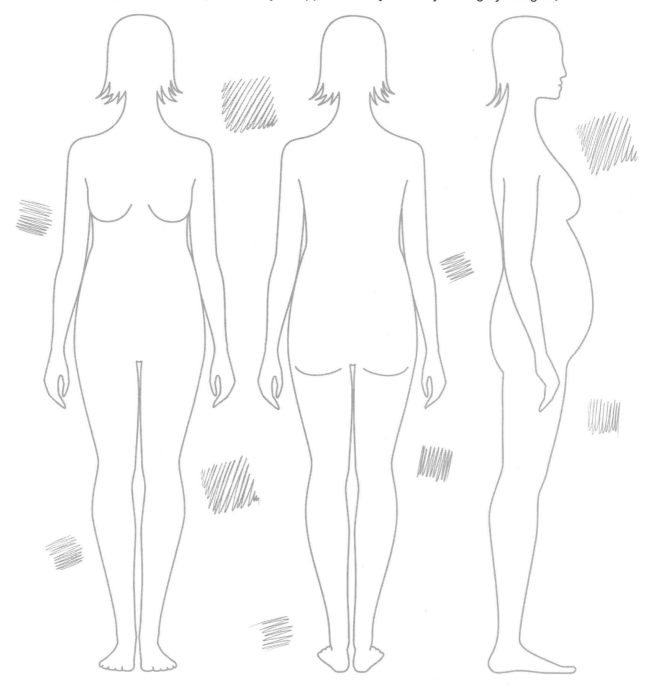

Meditation for Pregnant Zen

5, 6, 7, 8, let's all learn to meditate! Meditation can be super valuable to anyone—not just pregnant ladies. The host of benefits seem endless, so why not give it a go? Even taking just 10 minutes to meditate in the morning will boost your concentration and awareness throughout the rest of your day. Follow the steps below, and be patient.

1. Set Your Space

Dedicate a space in your home that is calm, quiet, and clean.

2. Set Your Time

Pick a time when your mind is calm. Most people meditate immediately upon waking up, or right before bedtime.

3. Set Your Routine

Use the same space and time for every meditation practice.

4. Get Comfy and Breathe

Sit with your back straight and your chin tilted slightly downward. Find additional support using a wall or pillow, if needed. Breathe deeply and regularly.

5. Let It Go

Make like Elsa, and let things (like intrusive thoughts) go. Acknowledge the thoughts that pop up, but don't attach to them. Allow them to pass by.

6. Focus

Focus on a specific point in the room. Or, close your eyes and hold an image in your mind's eye. Keep your focus but allow your mind to wander.

7. Meditate

Don't try to make it happen, it should be effortless.

8. Set Your Practice

Start with 10-minute sessions, then build up to the length of time that works best for you.

WTF Are You Thinking About Pie Chart: Second Trimester

It's time to visualize the many thoughts that are occupying your head. Fill out the pie chart below using the key and your own percentages.

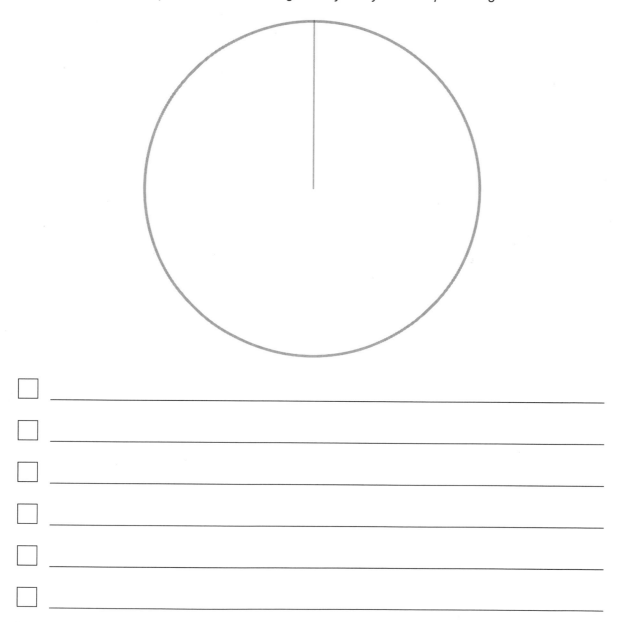

☐ _____

☐ _____

☐ _____

☐ _____

☐ _____

☐ _____

From Lemon to Lettuce: Second-Trimester Check-In

How are you feeling physically?

_____

_____

How are you feeling emotionally?

_____

_____

What are you thinking about frequently?

_____

_____

What are you excited for?

_____

_____

What are you nervous for?

_____

_____

What was one struggle you've overcome?

_____

_____

What was one of the best memories from this trimester?

_____

_____

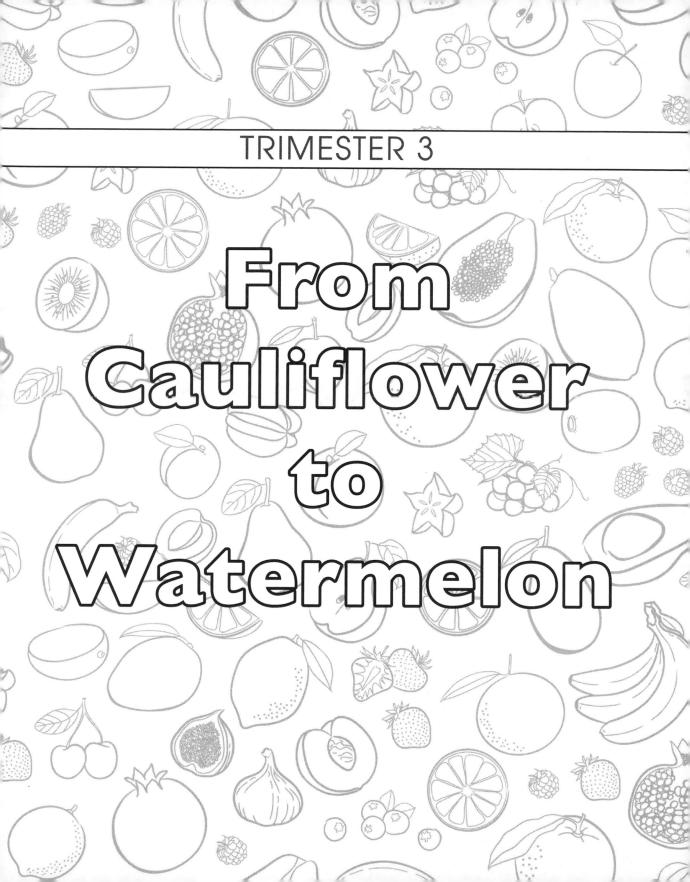

From Cauliflower to Watermelon

True or False: The Third-Trimester Edition

Last trimester! Do you know WTF is up with your body right now?
Focus that pregnancy brain of yours and get to quizzing.

1. Week 43 is when the baby is officially considered overdue. ❏ True ❏ False

2. Your baby's see-through skin becomes opaque during this time. ❏ True ❏ False

3. Your baby is starting to develop his or her first poop during the third trimester. ❏ True ❏ False

4. Your baby will be getting signals from all of his or her senses except for sight during the third trimester. ❏ True ❏ False

5. Dreaming. Your baby is doing it during the third trimester. ❏ True ❏ False

6. You will have sweet, peaceful dreams during this time. ❏ True ❏ False

7. Women tend to experience heartburn only during the third trimester. ❏ True ❏ False

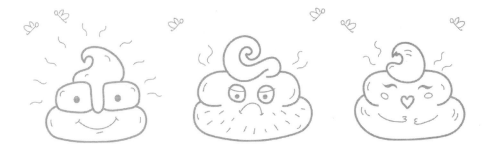

Answers on page 143.

Wish I could sleep, but someone is using my stomach for their own personal boxing gym!

Pre-Pregnancy vs. Current Favorite Outfits

*Draw what your favorite outfit was before you were pregnant,
and then draw your current favorite outfit.*

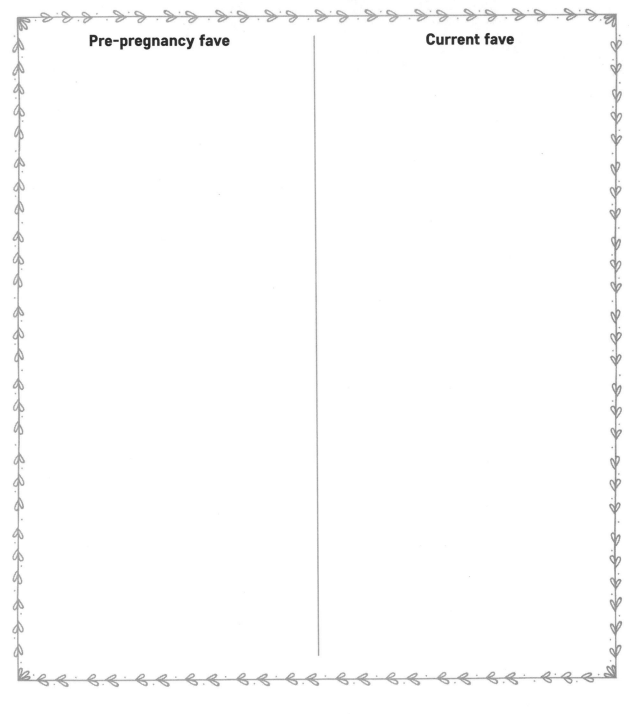

Pre-pregnancy fave   **Current fave**

How Many Words Can You Make?

How many words can you make out of the phrase:

She's about to pop?

Write them on the lines below.

_____ _____ _____

_____ _____ _____

_____ _____ _____

_____ _____ _____

_____ _____ _____

_____ _____ _____

_____ _____ _____

_____ _____ _____

_____ _____ _____

_____ _____ _____

_____ _____ _____

_____ _____ _____

_____ _____ _____

_____ _____ _____

_____ _____ _____

Sleeping Positions to Try

Hey, you probably aren't sleeping too great on account of how your organs are all squished and there's a karate kid punching your insides. Try these sleeping positions and see which one works best for you, and if none of them don't, well, it's not like you're ever going to sleep again anyways. Might as well get used to running on 57 minutes of shut-eye.

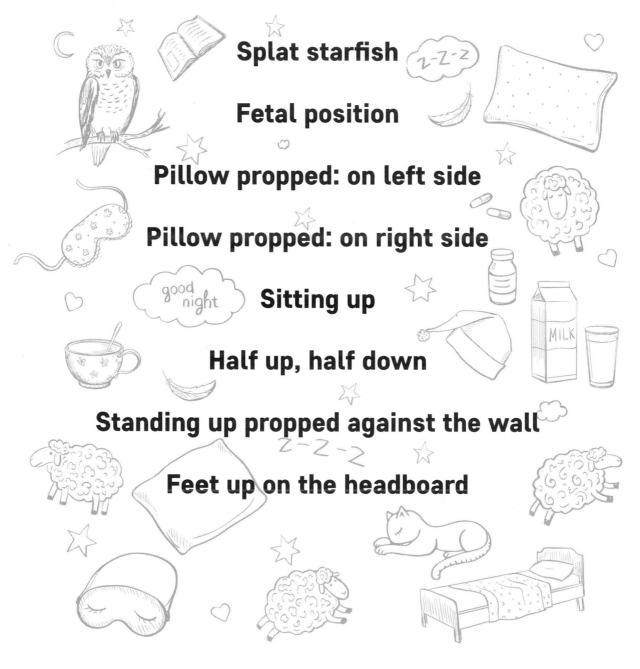

Splat starfish

Fetal position

Pillow propped: on left side

Pillow propped: on right side

Sitting up

Half up, half down

Standing up propped against the wall

Feet up on the headboard

Pack It Up Word Search

Oh, fuck! Your water broke and you have to pack your hospital bag in two minutes. How many essentials can you find in the word search? Circle the ones you find and cross them off the packing list. Can you find them all?

```
S  Q  D  L  Y  L  O  W  V  N  B  I  U  Y  H  L  B  G  W  J
B  J  E  W  W  C  S  D  R  K  C  O  B  W  N  S  A  A  B  R
S  E  H  T  O  L  C  Y  B  A  B  P  O  N  U  K  T  Z  S  E
C  R  E  G  R  A  H  C  M  B  T  P  O  J  K  E  H  B  U  T
P  O  R  T  A  B  L  E  S  P  E  A  K  E  R  W  T  H  L  R
J  U  M  S  N  A  C  K  S  C  U  C  E  B  R  K  O  C  T  W
L  F  K  F  R  W  Y  S  M  J  X  L  O  S  K  I  W  T  O  W
S  H  A  B  Y  H  R  J  C  H  D  T  G  E  R  B  E  L  E  N
Q  C  S  C  O  C  J  R  S  L  T  A  E  A  Q  A  L  G  X  I
E  N  O  U  E  J  L  U  K  L  E  T  T  D  J  I  C  P  G  B
E  L  H  I  R  W  R  O  E  J  A  Y  S  U  P  G  G  V  Q  B
J  A  R  M  Y  B  I  C  T  K  W  D  A  L  P  W  T  S  S  I
M  N  W  R  R  B  H  P  H  H  N  C  P  T  A  F  O  E  S  X
B  W  N  I  N  U  Z  T  E  N  E  T  H  D  U  K  J  L  F  V
G  X  A  I  M  M  U  I  O  S  W  S  T  I  L  E  I  T  R  M
W  H  C  L  U  F  Q  K  R  O  L  X  O  A  S  P  W  T  G  G
X  E  B  D  P  D  B  M  L  O  T  A  O  P  P  K  Q  O  W  O
D  E  O  D  O  R  A  N  T  U  B  X  T  E  B  E  P  B  T  C
S  C  T  I  G  C  J  A  A  N  G  E  R  R  F  Y  M  O  Y  A
Q  Z  N  K  P  C  G  E  U  I  H  S  W  S  J  T  V  B  O  G
```

Robe	Face wipes	Pillow	Baby clothes
Hair brush	Comfy clothes	Bath towel	Bottles
Toothbrush	Water bottle	Adult diapers	Snacks
Toothpaste	Slippers	Portable speaker	Book
Deodorant	Charger	Carseat	

Answers on page 144.

Sudoku Boredom Buster

				8	1			
8		3			9	7	1	
			4	3		9		5
4	7							1
3								9
5							3	2
7		8		1	4			
	2	5	6			1		8
			8	5				

Answers on page 144.

Poppin' Bottles Coloring Page

What you're about to be doing once you pop out that kid!

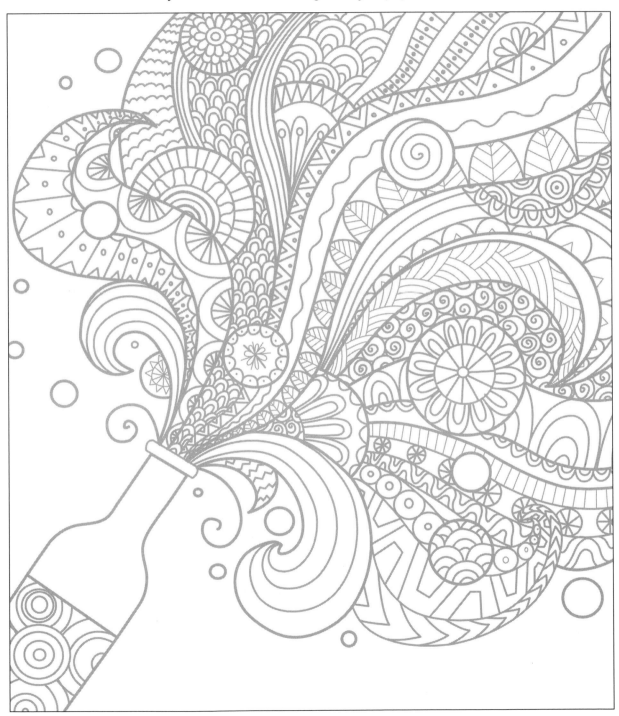

Uses for That Bump

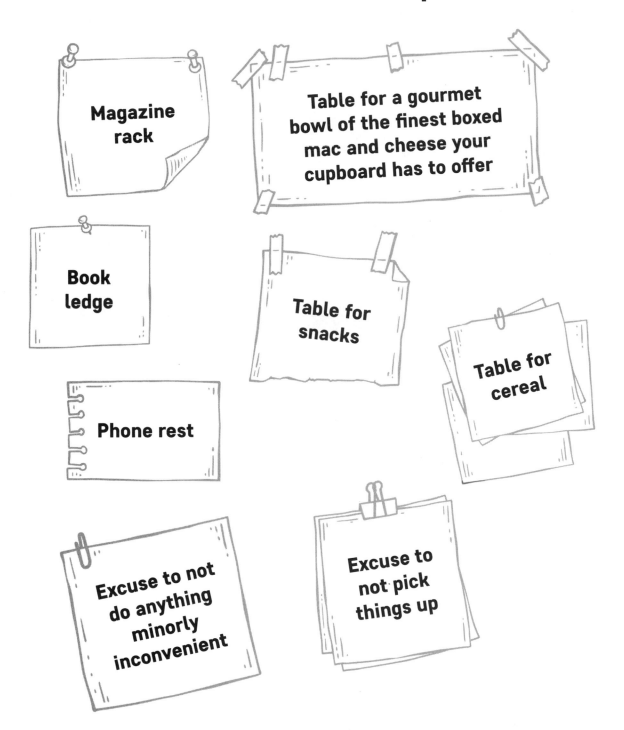

Magazine rack

Table for a gourmet bowl of the finest boxed mac and cheese your cupboard has to offer

Book ledge

Table for snacks

Table for cereal

Phone rest

Excuse to not do anything minorly inconvenient

Excuse to not pick things up

Drinking Game

No, not that kind of drinking game, unfortunately. How many cocktails that you're not allowed to have right now can you name in 30 seconds?

_____

_____

_____

_____

_____

_____

_____

_____

_____

_____

_____

_____

Lil Monster Coloring Page

Damn, girl, what are you growing in there? Mike Wazowski? Let's color in some lil monsters to honor the one that will soon be pooping and screaming in your arms (it's only a matter of time).

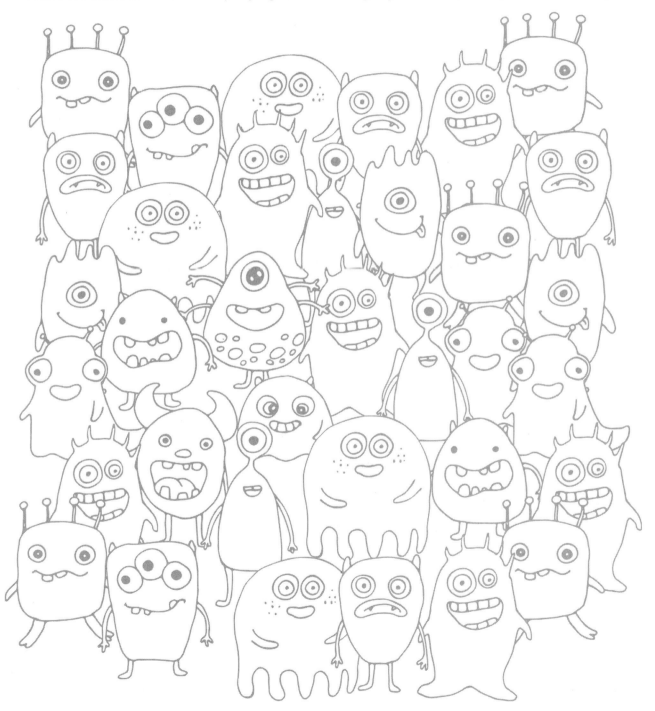

Anxiety-Busting Mandala Coloring Page

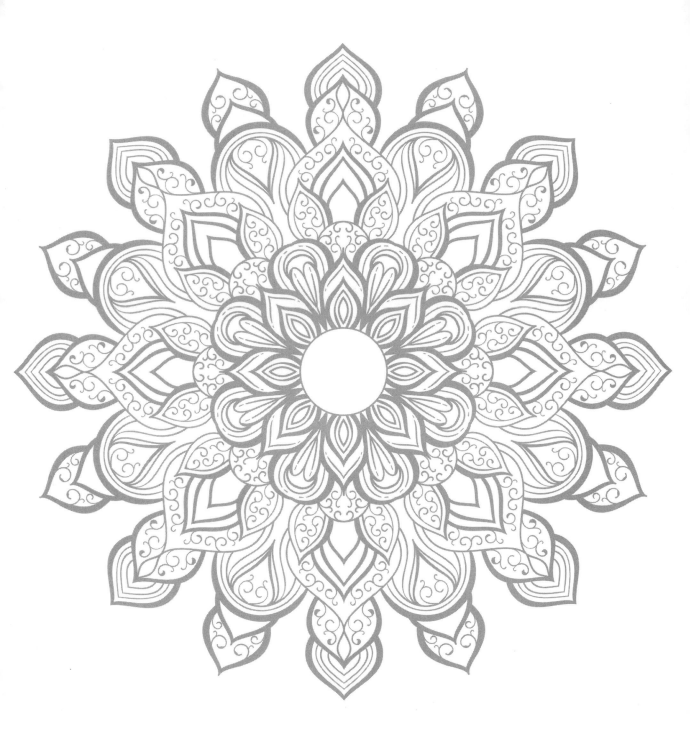

Find Your Way to the Hospital

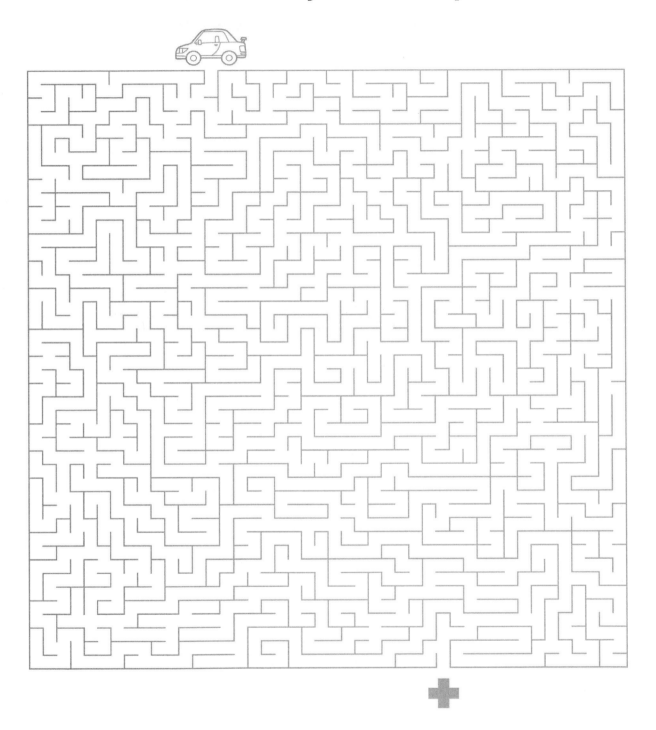

Answer on page 144.

Name That Kid from the Name of That Mom!

Here's a list of mom characters from various movies, TV shows, and books. How many of their kids can you name?

1. Coral _____

2. Sarabi _____

3. Helen Parr _____

4. Carol Brady _____

5. Lorelai Gilmore _____

6. Kitty Forman _____

7. Morticia Addams _____

8. Vivian Banks _____

9. Jane Jetson _____

10. Cersei Lannister _____

11. Marge Simpson _____

12. Bella Swan _____

13. Violet Crawley _____

14. Estelle Costanza _____

15. Molly Weasley _____

16. Samantha Stephens _____

17. Lucille Bluth _____

18. Marmee March _____

19. Ma Ingalls _____

Answers on page 144.

People always
say that
pregnant women
have a glow.
It's not a glow,
it's just sweat.

Things That Have Made You Go Apeshit

Have you ever seen a pregnant lady goin' apeshit? You might not be one of the Carters, but those pregnancy hormones can really make a person snap. List your top five apeshit moments below:

1. _____

_____

2. _____

_____

3. _____

_____

4. _____

_____

5. _____

_____

Decode the Message

Decode the secret message your baby is telling you when it kicks the shit out of your insides. Use the key provided:

.. / .- -- / .- .-.. -- --- ... -/ .-. . .- -.. -.-- /

– --- / -- . . –/ -.-- --- ..- / -- --- --

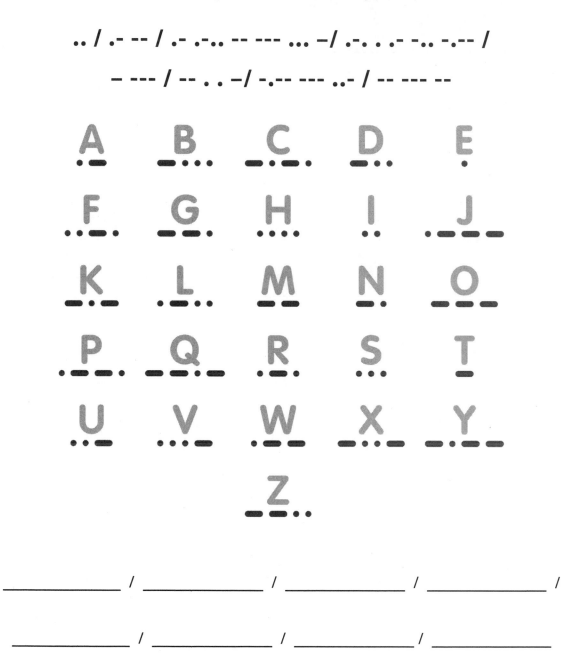

A ·—	B —···	C —·—·	D —··	E ·
F ··—·	G ——·	H ····	I ··	J ·———
K —·—	L ·—··	M ——	N —·	O ———
P ·——·	Q ——·—	R ·—·	S ···	T —
U ··—	V ···—	W ·——	X —··—	Y —·——
		Z ——··		

_____ / _____ / _____ / _____ /

_____ / _____ / _____ / _____

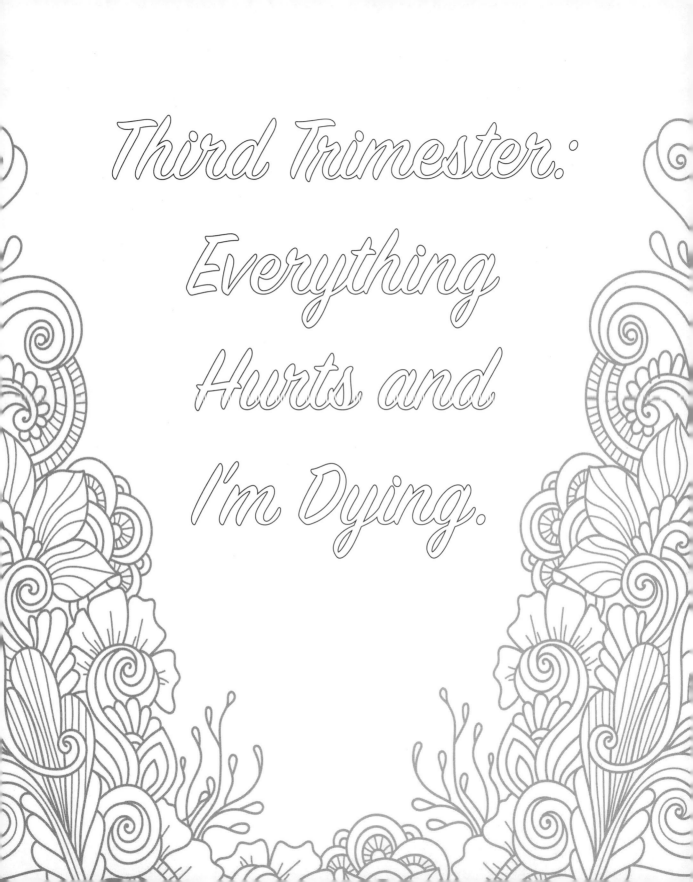

Third Trimester: Everything Hurts and I'm Dying.

Hospital Packing List

We know you've got a lot on your mind, so we've provided a basic packing list for the hospital trip, with some blank lines for adding anything else you might need.

❑ Photo ID

❑ Insurance information

❑ Hospital forms

❑ Birth plan (if you have one)

❑ Glasses (if you wear them)

❑ Contact lens case and solution

Toiletries:

❑ Hairbrush

❑ Toothbrush

❑ Toothpaste

❑ Deodorant

❑ Face wash

❑ Shampoo

❑ Conditioner

❑ Lotion

❑ Lip balm

❑ _____

❑ _____

❑ _____

❑ _____

❑ _____

Personal items:

❑ Cell phone

❑ Extension cord, phone charger, and portable phone charger

❑ Two or three pairs of warm, nonskid socks, unless you're fine using the hospital ones

❑ A warm robe or sweater you don't mind sacrificing to the cause

❑ Headband and ponytail holder

❑ Non-perishable snacks

❑ Two maternity bras (no underwire)

❑ Nursing pads

❑ _____

❑ _____

❑ _____

❑ _____

❑ _____

❑ _____

❑ _____

❑ _____

❑ _____

❑ _____

Fun Things to Do Now That You Can't See Your Feet

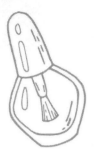
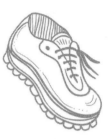

Drop things on the floor and leave them there

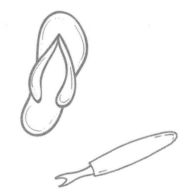

Make your partner cut your toenails

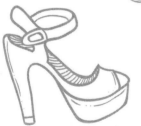

Hell, make your partner give you a full pedicure

Grow out your toe hairs and try to make a world record

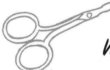

Wear mismatched shoes

Wear flip flops with socks

Lie down as much as possible to remind yourself that you have feet

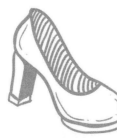
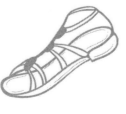
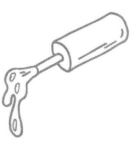

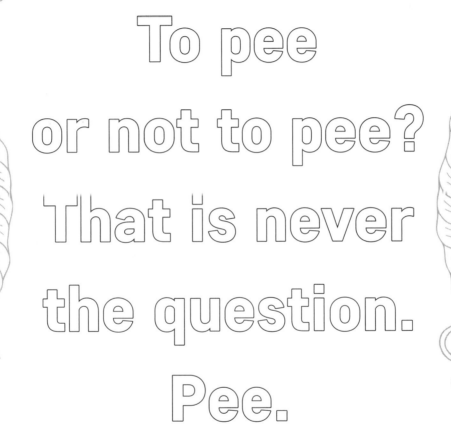

To pee
or not to pee?
That is never
the question.
Pee.

Your Final Form Coloring Page

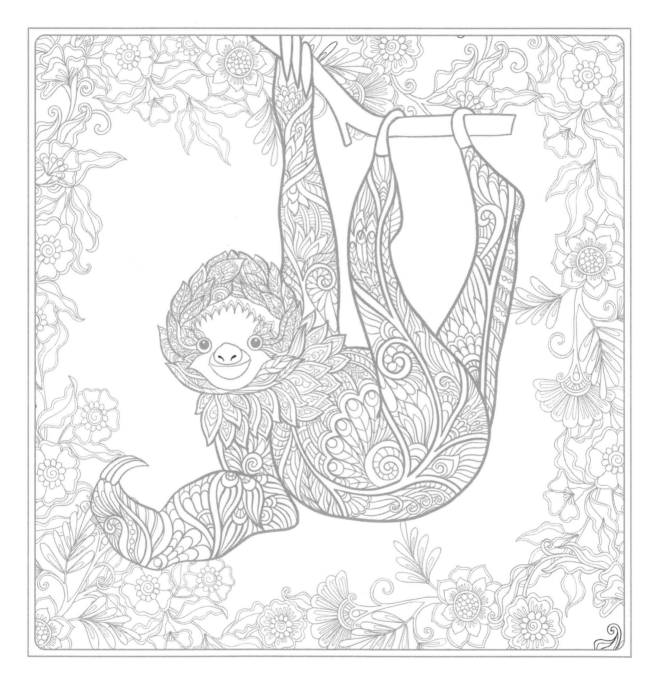

WTF Are You Thinking about Pie Chart: Third Trimester

What are you obsessing over during your third trimester?
Fill in the pie chart using the key and your own percentages.

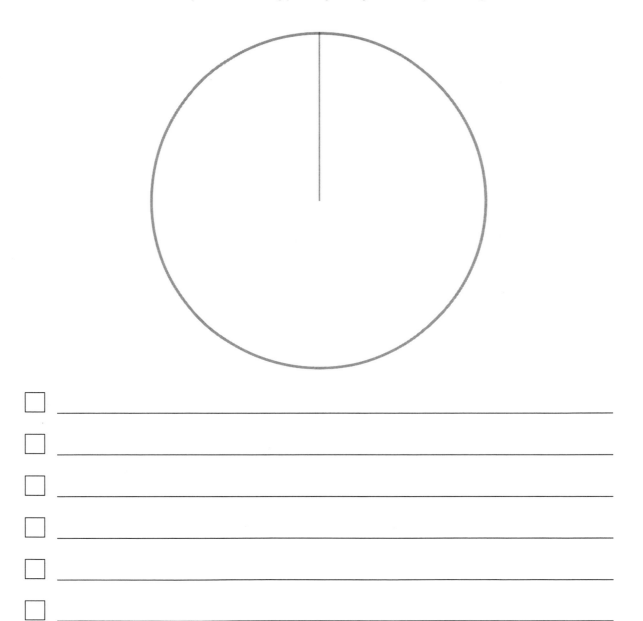

☐ _____

☐ _____

☐ _____

☐ _____

☐ _____

☐ _____

First Halloween Costume Quiz

Look it. Look it. It's freakin' bats. I love Halloween. What costume will you force your infant into, all in the name of spooky Halloween? Take the quiz to find out!

1. What is your favorite part of Halloween?

    A. The candy

    B. Looking at everyone's decorations

    C. Passing out candy to all the kiddos

    D. Haunted houses

2. What is your favorite Halloween movie?

    A. *Halloweentown*

    B. *Hocus Pocus*

    C. *Dracula*

    D. *Halloween*

3. What is your favorite candy?

    A. Reese's Peanut Butter Cups

    B. Classic Hershey's

    C. I like caramel apples better than candy.

    D. Candy corn

4. What face will you carve into your jack-o'-lantern?

    A. A smile

    B. A crescent moon and a witch on a broomstick

    C. I won't carve it, I'll just put the pumpkin out whole.

    D. The freakiest face I can create

5. What was your favorite Halloween costume as a child?

    A. A pumpkin

    B. A ghost

    C. A princess

    D. A witch

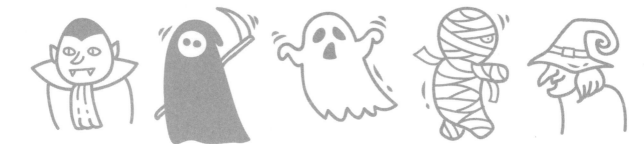

Mostly A's: A pot of spaghetti and meatballs

Mostly C's: Granny/Grandpa

Mostly B's: A freakin' bat

Mostly D's: Chuckie

Peezing:

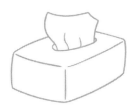

Verb. Sneezing and

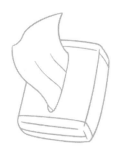

peeing at the

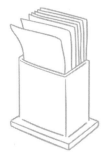

same time.

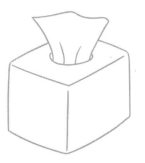

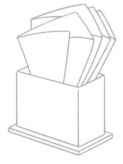

Journal Time

Third trimester, a time of near-constant freaking out. Let's take a moment to reflect on how you're feeling right at this moment and the things you're looking forward to once your baby comes.

_____

_____

_____

_____

_____

_____

_____

_____

_____

_____

_____

_____

_____

_____

_____

_____

Would You Rather: Celeb Baby Name Edition

If it's good enough for Kim K, it's good enough for you, peasant.

Gravity or Pilot Inspektor

_____ or Sunday Molly

_____ or Rocket

_____ or Cricket Pearl

_____ or Aleph

_____ or Bear Blu

_____ or Moroccan

_____ or Apple

_____ or Dusty Rose

_____ or North

_____ or Blue Ivy

_____ or Buddy Bear

_____ or Lazer

_____ or Diva Thin Muffin

_____ or Kal-El

_____ or Racer

_____ or Kulture

_____ or Reign

_____ or Saint

_____ or Petal Blossom Rainbow

_____ or Rumer

_____ or Fuschia

_____ or Elsie Otter

_____ or Moon Unit

We hope you chose Moon Unit as your final answer! If you didn't, you're wrong!

Unsolicited Advice Burn Book

Make a burn book of all the people who gave you unsolicited advice on how to give birth.

Name: _____

Unsolicited advice given: _____

_____

Name: _____

Unsolicited advice given: _____

_____

Name: _____

Unsolicited advice given: _____

_____

Name: _____

Unsolicited advice given: _____

_____

Name: _____

Unsolicited advice given: _____

_____

Name: _____

Unsolicited advice given: _____

_____

Refuel while Breastfeeding

If you choose to breastfeed your infant, you'll probably be burning around 500 calories a day! Damn! You'll need to stay full of good food to help your body replenish what that little vampire has sucked out. Color in the snacks that are a good idea and cross out the ones that are a bad idea.

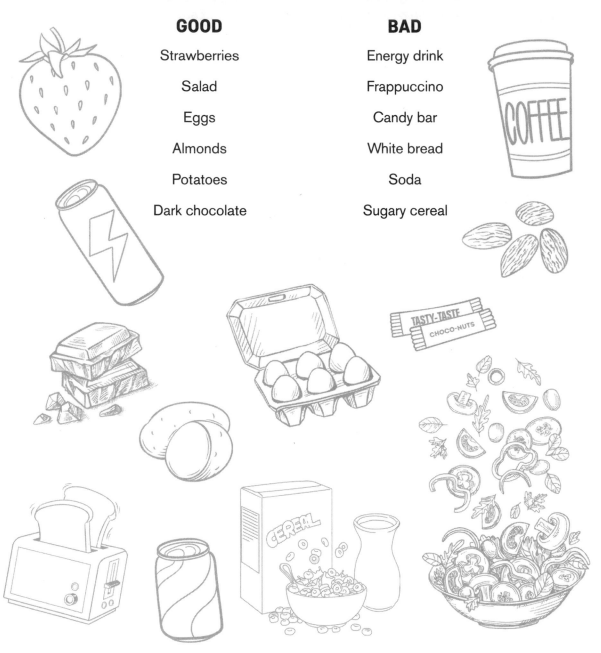

GOOD	BAD
Strawberries	Energy drink
Salad	Frappuccino
Eggs	Candy bar
Almonds	White bread
Potatoes	Soda
Dark chocolate	Sugary cereal

Mary Poppins Diaper Bag

It's time to make a list of all the things you're going to need in your never-ending magical carpet bag—er—your baby's diaper bag. We've given you a few suggestions to help things along.

☐ Traffic cones

☐ A lamp

☐ Another diaper bag

☐ A bottle of wine

☐ Ear plugs

☐ _____

☐ _____

☐ _____

☐ _____

☐ _____

☐ _____

☐ _____

☐ _____

☐ _____

☐ _____

☐ _____

☐ _____

☐ _____

☐ _____

☐ _____

☐ _____

☐ _____

☐ _____

☐ _____

☐ _____

☐ _____

☐ _____

☐ _____

☐ _____

☐ _____

☐ _____

☐ _____

☐ _____

☐ _____

Word Unscrambler

Unscramble the words and write them down in the spaces provided.

1. Folacrueilw _____

2. Nltaewmroe _____

3. Gnycnaerp _____

4. Ustef _____

5. Abby _____

6. Larpideu _____

7. Rlboa _____

8. Soicotrtnacn _____

9. Eemritstr _____

10. Wgiocrnn _____

Answers on page 144.

Pimp My Ride

Design your own ergonomic, aerodynamic, pimped AF stroller.
We've given you a base model to add onto.

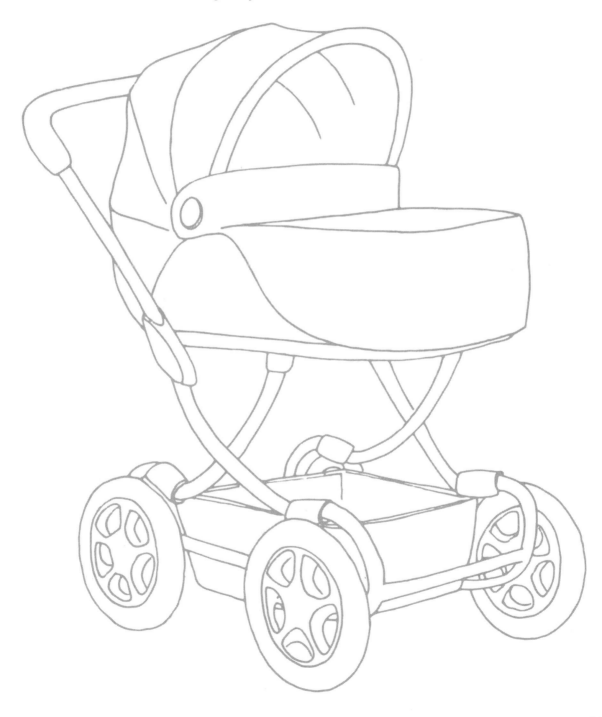

Quiz: What Theme Should You Have for Your Baby Shower?

Maybe you already have an idea for your baby shower, or maybe you haven't even begun to think about it. Regardless, we're here to help. Fill out the quiz and then use the key to find out what theme you should have for your baby shower.

1. What color combo do you like best?

A. Black and red

B. Teal and beige

C. Gold and white

D. Pink and green

2. Which decorations are a must-have?

A. Candles

B. Cute ones, like baby elephants and giraffes

C. Solo cups

D. Balloons, streamers, and flowers

3. What food would you serve?

A. The blood of your enemies

B. Sugar cookies

C. Jungle juice

D. Cupcakes and lemonade

4. What game would you play?

A. Guess the baby food

B. Don't Say "Baby"

C. Baby Bottle Chug

D. The Price Is Right—Baby Version

5. What gift do you hope to receive?

A. Anything black

B. Plushies

C. Alcohol for you to enjoy when you finally pop out this kid

D. Cute onesies

Mostly A's—Goth
Whoever said that a baby shower had to be all pastels and baby ducks? Deck the halls with black and red velvet and put on your darkest eyeliner. Light the candles and cue the organ—er, your playlist—and welcome your friends and family to the most hardcore baby shower they will ever attend.

Mostly B's—Animal Kingdom
What is almost as cute as the kid you're currently growing in your stomach? Baby animals, of course. Bring out your finest potted plants, hang up some adorable animal-themed decorations, and (if you really want to take things to the next level) have a face-painting station.

Mostly C's—Toga
Toga parties are not just for frat bros, bro. Why not throw a rager for your baby shower? It will certainly be a party to remember.

Mostly D's—Pinterest
Just go there and get your ideas.

A tie? Simply combine the two themes for an epically unique baby shower.

Circle the One That's Different

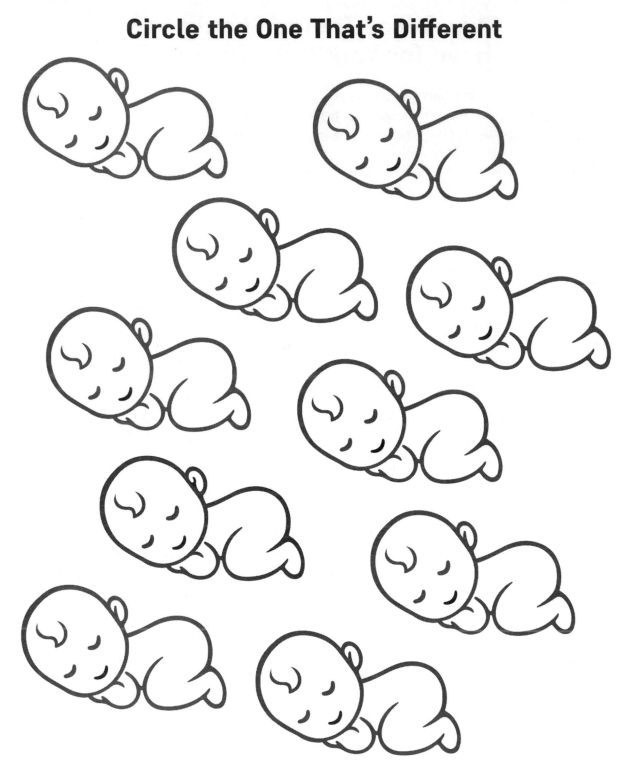

Answer on page 144.

OK I Really Need to Get This Thing Out of Me Right Now Checklist

Tired of feeling like you've got several bowling balls stuffed in your stomach? We feel ya. Though there is no one surefire way to encourage labor, here are some tips and tricks that have helped people in the past. Be sure to run everything by your doc before trying any of this at home!

Castor oil—A spoonful of castor oil is a treatment women have taken since times of yore. Though keep in mind that this nasty tasting oil is also used as a laxative, so be sure to stay hydrated if you decided to partake in this ye olde method.

Exercise—We're not saying to do one hundred burpees or a CrossFit class...just a walk will do. Try to get that heart rate up.

Acupuncture or pressure—Make an appointment and let someone else do the work. Even if it doesn't induce labor, you'll still feel the other benefits of these treatments.

A whole pineapple—Not proven to be effective, but hey, at least it's yummy.

Sex—Just get it on!

Herbal remedies—Drink red raspberry leaf tea during the days before your due date.

Nipple stimulation—Yep, you read that right.

Spicy food—This is an old wives' tale and certainly hasn't been proven. But if spicy foods are a part of your diet, there's no harm in continuing to eat them. If you are more of a "ketchup is spicy" kind of gal, maybe skip this one. You don't want to upset your stomach.

Things that you'd think would help but don't:
- Jumping jacks, jumping rope, pogo sticks, and other jumping-based activities
- Watching horror movies to scare the shit (and baby) out of you
- Giving that kid his or her first stern talking to
- Bargaining and/or bribing a higher power
- Complaining
- Packing and repacking your hospital bag
- Staring longingly at the empty crib

From Cauliflower to Watermelon:
Third-Trimester Check-In

How are you feeling physically?

_____

_____

How are you feeling emotionally?

_____

_____

What are you thinking about frequently?

_____

_____

What are you excited for?

_____

_____

What are you nervous for?

_____

_____

What was one struggle you've overcome?

_____

_____

What was one of the best memories from this trimester?

_____

_____

Letter to My Unborn Child

You certainly won't have time for this once you pop out that lil screamer, so let's get this over with now. Activate those pregnancy hormones and let's write out some sappy hopes and dreams for your sweet little babe!

_____

_____

_____

_____

_____

_____

_____

_____

_____

_____

_____

_____

_____

_____

_____

_____

_____

_____

_____

_____

_____

_____

_____

_____

_____

_____

_____

_____

_____

_____

_____

_____

Love,

Your mom _____

Answers

True or False: The First-Trimester Edition (page 8)

1. True, those lil chompers begin to form around week 6.

2. False, you technically conceive around week 2.

3. True. Heartbeats start around 5 weeks, and the earliest an ultrasound can detect pregnancy is at 5.5 weeks.

4. False, it has two.

5. True, you're basically growing a fish in there, lmao.

6. True, it's called parageusia and it can make even your fave beverage taste bad. Cheers, bitch!

Morning Sickness Word Search (page 14)

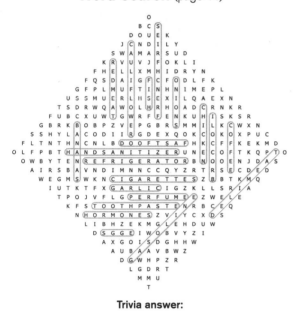

Trivia answer:
Hormones

I'm Fine with Water Crossword (page 18)

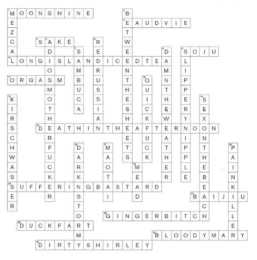

Sudoku Boredom Buster (page 22)

8	7	6	1	2	3	9	4	5
5	4	3	8	9	6	7	2	1
9	1	2	7	4	5	3	8	6
3	9	4	6	5	1	8	7	2
1	6	8	9	7	2	4	5	3
7	2	5	4	3	8	1	6	9
6	5	1	3	8	7	2	9	4
2	8	9	5	1	4	6	3	7
4	3	7	2	6	9	5	1	8

Pregnancy Symptoms Word Search (page 31)

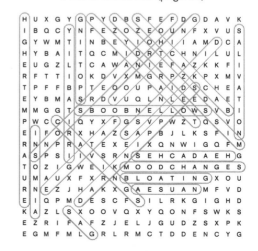

Pregnancy Cravings Word Search (page 32)

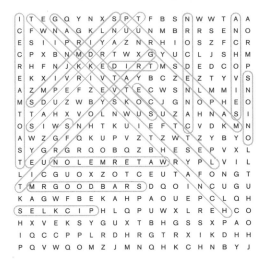

Baby Store Maze (page 40)

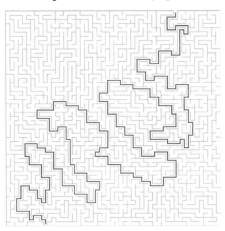

Nursery Rhyme Fill in the Blank (page 41)

1. fast
2. diamond
3. three
4. one
5. pail; tumbling
6. sheep's; cow's
7. contrary; silver; cockle
8. Drury Lane
9. rosie; posies
10. farmer's; tails; carving
11. curds; whey; spider

True or False: The Second-Trimester Edition (page 51)

1. True. This tends to happen toward week 20. Good thing you're pretty stretchy, lol!

2. False. On average, the fetus measures just up to 12 inches by the end of the second trimester. Still nothing to sneeze at!

3. True. Some days it'll feel like a soccer match up in there. GOOOOAALLLLL!

4. True. Bring some tissues wherever you go so you don't end up looking like Dracula.

5. False. Your boobs can still grow during the second trimester, and oftentimes one can be bigger than the other. Love that lopsided look!

6. True. This happens at around 22 weeks. Your baby definitely knows whether or not you're a terrible singer.

7. False, depending on the person. A lot of pregnant women report having pretty wild dreams during their second trimester, so strap the fuck in!

Nursery Word Search (page 52)

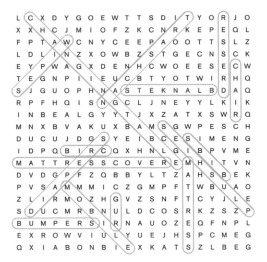

True or False: Let's Get Historical (page 58)

1. True. The beer was called groaning beer. Bottoms up, bitches.

2. False. In fact, taking pain-relieving herbs or draught during labor was forbidden (to the tune of being burned at the stake... yep) during the fifteenth and sixteenth centuries.

3. False. A widely popular sixteenth-century text, *The Rose Garden for Pregnant Women and Midwives*, written by Dr. Eucharius Rösslin, depicted fetuses as tiny adults floating around in the womb. Nice try, buddy.

4. True!

5. True: In the 1600s in France, up to five women used to share a maternity bed. Talk about unsanitary conditions!

6. False: Queen Victoria called for a pain-relieving drug during her childbirth in 1853, which paved the way for widespread acceptance.

7. False. C-sections were more likely named after the Latin word "caesuru," which means "to cut."

Lullaby Fill in the Blank (page 60)

1. tree top; rock, bough
2. mockingbird; mockingbird; diamond ring
3. sunshine; sunshine; gray; dear; sunshine
4. dilly, dilly; dilly, dilly

Sudoku Boredom Buster (page 64)

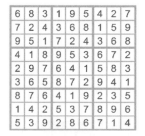

Avoid-the-Unwarranted-Advice Maze (page 67)

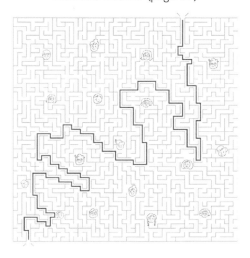

Match It Up! (page 70)

William—With gilded helmet

Benjamin—Son of my right hand

Caleb—Whole hearted

Oliver—Descendant of the ancestor

Wyatt—Brave in war

Chidi—God exists

Daisuke—Large, great

Sheng—Victory

Apu—Pure, virtuous, divine

Enrique—Home ruler

Nora—Honor

Margot—Pearl

Abigail—Joy of the father

Lucy—Light

Penelope—With a Web over her face

Kamili—Perfection

Inari—Successful one

Mei—Plum

Bhavna—Good feelings

Esperanza—Hope

Mom Unscrambler (page 76)

1. Leonardo DiCaprio
2. Kim Kardashian
3. *Frozen*
4. Robert De Niro
5. *Ocean's 13*
6. Reese Witherspoon
7. *Lady Bird*
8. *Mamma Mia*

Science Rules Crossword Puzzle (page 80)

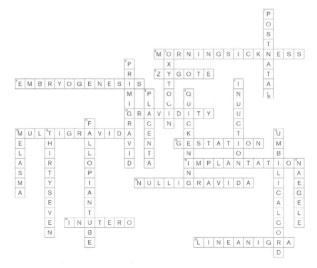

True or False: The Third-Trimester Edition (page 94)

1. False. It's week 42.

2. True.

3. True, mostly within the final weeks. How adorably gross!

4. False. Your baby will get signals from all five senses.

5. True.

6. True. Time to do those Kegels, ladies!

7. False. Women also experience heartburn during the second trimester, but it's during the third when your jam-packed uterus pushes your stomach (and whatever pregnancy cravings you've recently eaten) upward. Uncomfy!

Pack It Up Word Search (page 99)

```
S Q D L Y L O W V N B I U Y H L B G W J
B J E W W C S D R K C O B W N S A A B R
S E H T O L C Y B A B P O N U K T Z S E
C R E G R A H C M B T P O J K E H B U T
P O R T A B L E S P E A K E R W T H L R
J U M S N A C K S C U C E B R K O C T W
L F K F R W Y S M J X L O S K I W T O W
S H A B Y H R J C H D T G E R B E L E N
Q C S C O C J R S L T A E A N L G X I
E N O U E J L U K L E T T D J I C P G B
E L H I R W R O E J A Y S U P G G V Q B
J A R M Y B I C T K W D A L P W T S S I
M N W R R B H P H N C P T A F O E S X
B W N I N U Z T E N E T H D U K J L F V
G X A I M M U I O S W S T I L E I T R M
W H C L U F Q K R O L X O A S P W T G G
X E B D P D B M L O T A O P P K Q O W O
D E O D O R A N T U B X T E B E P B T C
S C T I G C J A A N G E R R F Y M O Y A
Q Z N K P C G E U I H S W S J T V B O G
```

Sudoku Boredom Buster (page 100)

6	5	9	7	8	1	3	2	4
8	4	3	5	2	9	7	1	6
2	1	7	4	3	6	9	8	5
4	7	2	3	9	8	5	6	1
3	8	1	2	6	5	4	7	9
5	9	6	1	4	7	8	3	2
7	6	8	9	1	4	2	5	3
9	2	5	6	7	3	1	4	8
1	3	4	8	5	2	6	9	7

Find You Way to the Hospital (page 109)

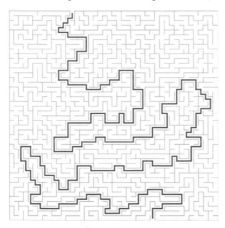

Name That Kid from the Name of That Mom (page 110)

1. Nemo
2. Simba
3. Violet, Dash, and Jack-Jack Parr
4. Greg, Peter, Bobby, Marcia, Jan, and Cindy
5. Rory Gilmore
6. Laurie and Eric Forman, and Steven Hyde (foster son)
7. Wednesday and Pugsley Addams
8. Nicky, Ashley, Carlton, and Hillary Banks
9. Judy and Elroy Jetson
10. Joffrey, Myrcella, and Tommen Baratheon (and an unnamed son, fathered by Robert Baratheon)
11. Bart, Lisa, and Maggie Simpson
12. Renesmee Carlie Cullen
13. Rosamund and Robert
14. George Costanza
15. Fred, George, Ron, Charlie, Ginny, Bill, and Percy Weasley
16. Tabitha and Adam Stephens
17. George Michael Bluth
18. Meg, Jo, Beth, and Amy March
19. Mary, Laura, Caroline, Charles "Freddie," and Grace Ingalls

Word Unscrambler (page 132)

1. Cauliflower
2. Watermelon
3. Pregnancy
4. Fetus
5. Baby
6. Epidural
7. Labor
8. Contractions
9. Trimester
10. Crowning

Circle the One That's Different (page 136)

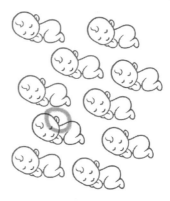